Praise for *Change Your Environments*

"If you are like most people, you are overwhelmed with the full-time, even around-the-clock, job that just living life and staying healthy has become. Microplastics, pesticides, mercury, don't eat this or that, ultra-processed foods . . . What should you believe and how can you distill it down to truly manageable strategies before you throw your hands up in frustration? In *Change Your Environments*, Dr. Berg brings his signature straight-talking style and provides a virtual GPS for navigating all the complexities and nuances of these issues, providing clear, straightforward advice that even your teenager can manage."

—William Davis, MD, #1 *New York Times* bestselling author of *Wheat Belly*, *Super Gut*, and *Super Body*

"In *Change Your Environments*, Dr. Eric Berg offers a practical and thought-provoking framework for understanding how our daily surroundings shape our health. The book reminds us that many of the most powerful health interventions are not complicated. Whether it is spending more time outdoors, improving sleep, reducing environmental stressors, or redesigning daily habits, Dr. Berg provides a roadmap for creating conditions in which health can flourish. It is a timely reminder that sometimes the path to better health begins not with adding something new, but with reconnecting to what has been there all along."

—Roger Seheult, MD

"Some health care experts are good at theory and have a great knowledge of the literature of health and medicine, but what they know is through the eyes and experience of others. Dr. Berg is no such doctor. He gets down into the nitty gritty of food and environmental control, and the living dirt on his farms to really *know* what he is talking about because he has lived it and is doing it, and then as a master teacher, communicating these principles, so others can learn them and live them. In this book, you will understand the essential tools to live healthy and long. What better gift could an author give?"

—David I. Minkoff, MD

"As a heart surgeon, I see every day how the environments we live in drive the metabolic disease that lands patients on my operating table. Dr. Eric Berg's *Change Your Environments* gives you the missing map: nine key environments, a simple audit to identify your highest-leverage fixes, and the insight that improving one upstream environment creates powerful cascading improvements in the others. This is the practical redesign tool that finally makes sustainable metabolic health achievable—without needing more willpower."

—Philip Ovadia, MD, author of *Stay Off My Kitchen Table*

"In my work helping patients reverse diabetes, I see firsthand that chronic metabolic issues aren't a failure of willpower. Your hormones are simply reacting to a chaotic modern lifestyle. In *Change Your Environments*, Dr. Berg skips useless band-aids like calorie counting and focuses entirely on fixing the spaces where we live and work. By changing the simple inputs around you, you let your body naturally reset your blood sugar, sleep, and weight. It's a practical, real-world guide that gets straight to the root cause."

—Dr. Roshani Sanghani, endocrinologist and author of *Turn Around Diabetes: A Step-by-Step Guide*

"For thirty years I watched patients arrive with a drawer full of single answers: one pill, one diet, one exercise that was going to fix everything. It almost never did, because health is not a single problem to be solved. It is many connected systems, and you cannot repair one while the others keep doing damage. This book is the first I have seen that addresses the whole picture and provides an actionable, easy-to-follow map. Specific steps, no generalities. It shows you where your own weak point is and exactly what to do about it. A must-read."

—Dr. Dimitris Tsoukalas, MD, PhD,
founder of Metabolomic Medicine® Clinics

CHANGE YOUR ENVIRONMENTS

Redesign Your Life to Reclaim Your Health

ERIC BERG, DC

MAHA
BOOKS

MAHA Books may be purchased in bulk at special discounts for sales promotion, corporate gifts, fund-raising, or educational purposes. Special editions can also be created to specifications. For details, contact the Special Sales Department, Skyhorse Publishing, 307 Fifth Avenue, 4th Floor, New York, NY 10016 or info@skyhorsepublishing.com.

MAHA Books is an imprint of Skyhorse Publishing, Inc.®, a Delaware corporation.

Visit our website at www.skyhorsepublishing.com.

Please follow our publisher Tony Lyons on Instagram @tonylyonsisuncertain.

10 9 8 7 6 5 4 3 2 1

Library of Congress Control Number: 2026946204

Cover design by Brian Peterson

Print ISBN: 978-1-63144-119-6
Ebook ISBN: 978-1-63144-120-2

Printed in the United States of America

To all of you who live on planet Earth—an environment that won't let you win. Until now.

Contents

Acknowledgments

This book began with the patients I couldn't stop thinking about—not the ones who got better, but the ones who did everything right and still couldn't get traction. Those are the ones I drove home thinking about, for years. Over more than forty years they taught me the same lesson, again and again, until I finally listened: The problem was almost never the person. It was the environment around them. Whatever is useful in these pages, they are the reason I went looking for it.

And then there's my wife, Karen—my chief guinea pig and the most patient person I know. For years I've come to her with the same opening line: "Honey, I've got another idea I want to try." She gives me a look, says, "Oh boy—here we go again," and then rolls up her sleeves and tries it with me anyway. A good deal of what I've learned about changing an environment, I learned by changing ours—usually before breakfast, usually without much warning. None of this would exist without her patience, her honesty, and her willingness to let our home be what we call the sandbox.

BEFORE WE BEGIN

Why I Wrote This Book

I've been helping people with their health for a long time.

For more than thirty years—first in private practice, and then as a health educator with one of the largest platforms on the Internet—I've seen a lot of different patients, for a lot of different problems. And I've helped a lot of people. For most of my career, I did it by focusing on the questions most doctors focus on, but using natural methods: What's the best remedy for this symptom?

Results were hit or miss.

But I'll tell you what bugged me. I'd go home at night, and the patients I'd find myself thinking about weren't the ones who got better. They were the few who didn't. The ones who couldn't quite change their ways—or who changed them for a while, fell off the wagon, and couldn't get back on. Those are the ones my attention got stuck on. For years.

Over time, I transitioned into asking why—and digging deeper into the root causes.

And I stumbled onto the best way to diagnose—or really, to figure out—a person's health problem. It's actually well studied; there's a whole science, with textbooks, wrapped around it.

What I've done is build a framework around nine specific environments—food, light and sleep, movement, chemical, microbiome, cognitive-dopamine, social, workspace, and nutrients. These are the nine zones of your life that your body is in constant conversation with, whether you're paying attention or not.

Most health books give you a method. This one gives you a map. The method tells you what to do. The map tells you where your problem actually lives—so you stop fixing the wrong thing.

That map has a name: ancestral mismatch. It's the gap between the environment your body was built for—the one it spent two and a half million years adapting to—and the modern one it's actually living in. When I scan through those nine environments with a patient and find the greatest mismatch, I've found the root cause. Every time.

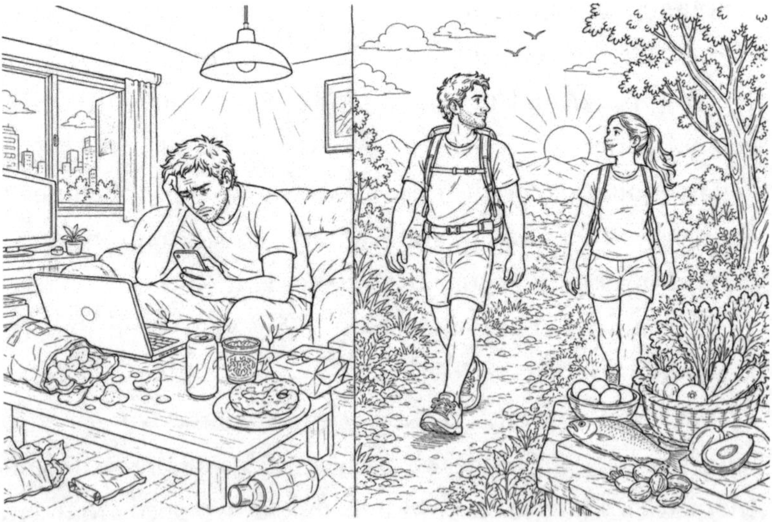

What I've done in this book is take that diagnostic lens and turn it into a redesign tool. Not "eat less, move more." Not a better mindset. A different environment—in nine specific places where your biology is currently getting the wrong information.

This book is that framework.

How the Nine Environments Talk to Each Other

Here's something important before you start.

These nine environments are not nine separate problems. They are one system. And they talk to each other constantly.

A broken food environment raises insulin and drives inflammation—which degrades your sleep architecture, which raises cortisol, which increases cravings the next day, which makes the food environment harder to fix. A chemical environment overloaded with endocrine disruptors disrupts hormonal signaling—which destabilizes your microbiome, which impairs neurotransmitter production, which makes your cognitive-dopamine environment fragile, which makes every other change harder to sustain.

One broken environment cascades. But cascades run both ways—and this is the part that changes everything.

Fix one environment at the source, and the ones downstream of it start improving on their own—without you touching them directly. Fix your food timing, and your sleep improves without touching your sleep environment. Fix your light environment, and your next-day food cravings drop—because poor sleep drives ghrelin up and leptin down, and your body is asking for sugar before you've made a single choice. Fix your movement environment, and your stress hormone burden drops, and your microbiome diversifies, and your cognitive environment gets sharper.

You are not managing nine independent problems. You are redesigning one system—and every fix you make creates leverage in places you didn't directly touch.

That's why this book works when willpower alone doesn't. Willpower fights one craving at a time. Environment redesign changes the conditions that produce the craving. You're not pushing the boulder uphill. You're tilting the hill.

Here's a simple map of the biggest cascade relationships—so you can see where your leverage is highest:

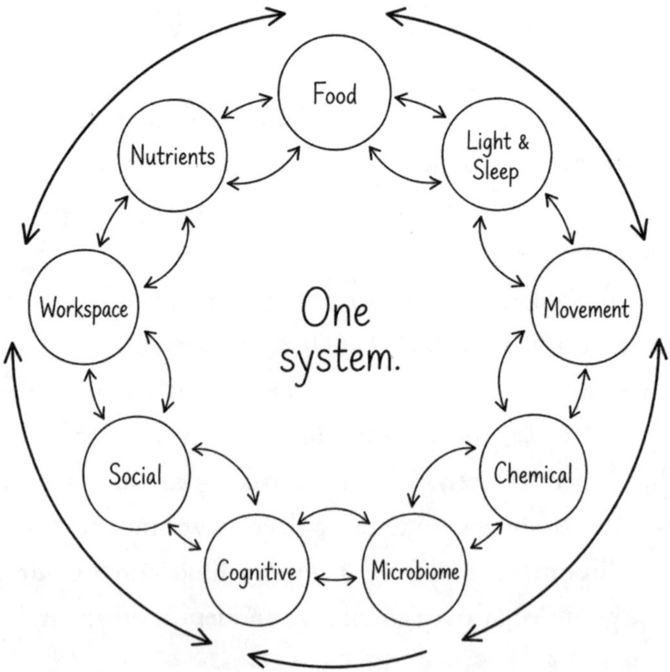

If this environment is broken . . .	It typically damages . . .
Food	Sleep quality, microbiome diversity, cognitive-dopamine
Light & Sleep	Food cravings, movement energy, hormone balance
Chemical	Microbiome, hormone signaling, sleep quality
Movement	Stress hormone load, cognitive function, sleep depth
Microbiome	Immune function, cognitive-dopamine, chemical clearance
Cognitive-Dopamine	Food environment, social behavior, workspace focus
Social	Cognitive-dopamine, stress load, movement motivation
Workspace	Movement patterns, cognitive function, sleep posture
Nutrients	All systems—foundational to every other environment

You'll notice the connections as you read. I'll point them out at the end of each chapter. And once you've done the audit and found your two most broken environments—start there. Fix the upstream ones first. Let the cascade work for you.

Now, why did all nine of these environments break at the same time? There's one answer.

Because here's the hidden step almost nobody tells you about. We are living in a very strange modern environment—one that is nothing like what the body was actually designed for. It has been engineered for addiction, for comfort, for abundance. You can order food and have it delivered around the clock. You barely have to expend any energy at all—a few steps to the fridge or the pantry, and presto, instant snacks.

Changing your environments also ends the constant need

for more willpower and discipline. You reorganize things so there's less friction for the good habits, and added friction for the bad ones.

This is what's behind the New Year's resolution that lasts all of a few weeks. Why? Because you never changed your environment. So as soon as life—stress—kicks in, the willpower goes right out the window.

You can go ahead and try to fight that with discipline. Some people succeed. But most fall off the wagon. When you're tired, stressed, or bored, your body will override your good intentions without much trouble at all—as long as the easy, engineered option is sitting right there, available, at exactly that moment.

And it really is your body that overrides your willpower, because our surroundings have been so highly engineered for addiction.

So this book is written for the person who has tried, and tried, and tried. The person who is not lazy, not uninformed, and not unwilling to do the work. The person who has followed the advice and still isn't where they want to be—and who suspects, correctly, that the real problem isn't something they're doing wrong, but something sitting deeper.

I think you'll be pleasantly surprised—this is finally going to work for you. The days of "just try harder" are over.

I'm not going to ask you to try harder, or change your mindset, or have better self-control. I'm only going to help you redesign all nine environments, one by one. Take your time, and let them compound.

I want to lessen your choices—so the only ones left are the healthy ones.

You do not need more willpower. You need better environments.

Let's build them.

—Eric Berg, DC
Alexandria, Virginia, 2026

The Environment Audit

Find Your Starting Point

Before you read another word, take ten minutes and do this. Your results will tell you which chapters to read first—and which single change is likely to unlock the most.

Prefer to do this online? Take the same assessment as the Health Lever Quiz at drberg.com/health-lever-quiz—same questions, instant results.

This is not a medical test. It maps your **environment**—the inputs and surroundings you can redesign—not a diagnosis. (See the note on evidence at the end.)

How to Score

For each statement, choose the number that fits right now:

- **2**—Yes / true most days
- **1**—Somewhat / a few days a week / partly true
- **0**—No / rarely or never true

Each section has five statements, so each section scores **0–10**. Write your number next to each statement, total each section, then carry your totals to the scoring page.

Every statement describes your *environment or routine*, not how you feel. (There's a separate, optional feelings check at the end—don't fold it into these scores.)

ENVIRONMENT 1: FOOD

1. Ultra-processed snacks—chips, crackers, cookies, candy—are kept within easy reach at home or work.
2. My eating is spread across the day with no consistent start-and-stop window.
3. The drinks I reach for by default carry calories or sugar—soda, juice, sports drinks, sweetened coffee.
4. There are few visible, grab-and-go whole foods where I live—fruit, cut veg, boiled eggs, plain nuts.
5. I usually eat while distracted—at a screen, a desk, or driving—rather than at a table.

Section 1 total: ___ / 10

ENVIRONMENT 2: LIGHT & SLEEP

6. I don't get outdoors into natural daylight within about thirty minutes of waking.
7. My bedroom isn't fully dark at night—standby LEDs, streetlight, or a charging phone.
8. I use screens within two to three hours of going to sleep.
9. My wake-up time swings by more than about 30–60 minutes across the week.
10. I have caffeine—coffee, tea, energy drinks—past early afternoon.

Section 2 total: ___ / 10

ENVIRONMENT 3: MOVEMENT

11. I sit for stretches of 60+ minutes with nothing built in to get me up.
12. My day has no built-in walking—daily destinations aren't within walking reach.
13. My surroundings make driving the automatic choice even for short trips.
14. There's no standing or movement option set up where I work—no standing desk, no cue to get up.
15. My only real activity is one workout; the rest of the day defaults to sitting.

Section 3 total: ___ / 10

ENVIRONMENT 4: CHEMICAL

This is the most scientifically contested section—see the evidence note. Treat high scores as "worth a low-cost swap," not alarm.

16. I cook on scratched or worn nonstick cookware.
17. I microwave or pour hot food into plastic containers.
18. My everyday personal-care products are heavily scented—"fragrance" or "parfum" high on the label.
19. My drinking water sits in plastic that gets warm—bottles in a hot car, garage, or sunlight.
20. Scented air products run regularly in my space—plug-ins, sprays, or frequent scented candles.

Section 4 total: ___ / 10

ENVIRONMENT 5: MICROBIOME

21. I rarely eat a variety of deeply colored, polyphenol-rich vegetables—the kind that feed beneficial gut microbes.
22. I'm currently a regular user of a gut-disrupting medication—frequent antibiotics, a daily acid-blocker, or near-daily NSAIDs (ibuprofen).
23. Fermented foods are essentially absent from my week—yogurt, kefir, sauerkraut, kimchi.
24. Gluten and refined-grain foods are a regular part of my diet—bread, pasta, cereal, baked goods—the staples that damage the gut lining.
25. Synthetic food additives are regular in my diet—artificial sweeteners, emulsifier-heavy packaged foods.

Section 5 total: ___ / 10

ENVIRONMENT 6: COGNITIVE

26. My phone is always within reach—no phone-free zones or times exist in my day.
27. My work setup keeps messaging, social, or news one click away while I'm trying to focus.
28. Push notifications are on for many apps, so my phone interrupts me through the day.
29. My phone is the first thing I touch in the morning and the last at night—it's within reach of the bed.
30. My recreational screen time runs to roughly two hours or more on a typical day.

Section 6 total: ___ / 10

ENVIRONMENT 7: SOCIAL

The people, patterns, and structures around you that either support or drain your biology.

31. My week rarely includes unhurried, in-person conversation that isn't about work, errands, or logistics.
32. Someone I'm regularly around leaves me feeling criticized, undermined, or small.
33. There's no one in my life I can be completely honest with about what's really going on.
34. My living or working setup leaves me isolated for long stretches by default.
35. Most of my obligatory social contact is with people who drain rather than restore me.

Section 7 total: ___ / 10

ENVIRONMENT 8: WORKSPACE

36. My main screen sits below eye level, so I look or hunch downward at it.
37. My workspace is noisy or interrupt-prone in ways I can't control.
38. My workspace gets no natural daylight and no sightline to rest my eyes at a distance.
39. The air in my workspace feels stale—windows don't open, no plants, ventilation unchecked.
40. I work in the same space where I rest or sleep, with no boundary between them.

Section 8 total: ___ / 10

ENVIRONMENT 9: NUTRIENTS

This overlaps Food and Microbiome by nature. It's aimed narrowly at a few micronutrients that food quantity doesn't guarantee.

41. I get little sun on my skin and rarely eat vitamin-D foods (oily fish, fortified foods)—so my D intake is likely low.
42. Magnesium-rich foods and waters are rare in my week—leafy greens, avocado, dark chocolate (low sugar), and mineral-rich spring, well, or mineral water.
43. I eat oily fish (salmon, sardines, mackerel) fewer than about twice a week and have no other omega-3 source.
44. Most of my calories come from refined or processed foods stripped of their vitamins and minerals.
45. My diet has run the same for years with no check—bloodwork, a clinician, a dietitian—on whether it's meeting my needs.

Section 9 total: ___ / 10

Scoring Your Results

Add up each section. Your total possible is 90. The higher a number, the more that environment is working against you.

What Each Section Score Means

Section score	Priority	What it means
7–10	Critical	A broken environment. Start here.
4–6	Compromised	Holding you back. Get to it after the critical ones.
0–3	Functioning	Doing okay. Read the chapter to fine-tune.

Where to Start

Find your **single highest-scoring section** and go to that chapter first. If two or more sections tie—or once your top one is underway and you have room for a second—use this tie-break: **start with the one whose "Start Here" move is easiest for you to do this week.** Early momentum matters more than rank order.

Section	Chapter
1. Food	Chapter 1
2. Light & Sleep	Chapter 2
3. Movement	Chapter 3
4. Chemical	Chapter 4
5. Microbiome	Chapter 5
6. Cognitive	Chapter 6
7. Social	Chapter 7
8. Workspace	Chapter 8
9. Nutrients	Chapter 9

What Your Total Means

Total 0–18—Largely working. You're fine-tuning, not rebuilding. Read any chapter in any order.

Total 19–36—A few rough spots. Two or three environments are dragging on each other. Order matters: Fix your highest-scoring section first and the others tend to ease.

Total 37–54—Several broken. This is common for people who feel like they're doing everything right and getting nowhere. The problem usually isn't willpower—it's architecture. Start with your single highest section. Don't try to fix everything at once.

Total 55–90—Most things out of step. That's not a character flaw—it's a design problem, and you can redesign an environment faster than you can build a habit. Take your top three sections and start with just the Start Here move in each.

The Pattern to Watch For

These are *examples* of common clusters, not the only ones. The general rule underneath them: When your top sections share an upstream driver, start with the section that feeds the others.

- **Top scores in Food, Cognitive, and Light & Sleep (1, 6, 2):** These tend to feed each other—late screens and irregular eating disturb sleep, and short sleep drives the next day's cravings and screen-pull. **Likely highest-leverage start: Chapter 2 (Light & Sleep)**, because fixing light and timing often steadies the whole loop.
- **Top scores in Chemical, Microbiome, and Nutrients (4, 5, 9):** These often chain together—but this is also the most evidence-thin trio, so treat it as low-cost swaps. **A reasonable start: Chapter 4 (Chemical)** to reduce easy-to-remove inputs, then rebuild the gut in Chapter 5.

- **Top scores in Movement, Cognitive, and Social (3, 6, 7):** Too much sitting and too little connection both add low-grade stress that keeps mood and focus foggy. **Often the fastest relief: Chapter 3 (Movement).**

The general move: Look at your two or three highest sections and ask which one, if fixed, would make the others easier. Start there.

Optional: A Feelings Baseline

How you feel is an *outcome*, not an environment—so it's deliberately kept out of the scoring above. But it's worth a quick baseline so you can tell whether your changes are working. Tick anything that's been true lately, note the date, and recheck in a few weeks once you've started on your top section:

- Shaky, foggy, or irritable if I go a few hours without eating
- Strong, hard-to-ignore sugar or refined-carb cravings most days
- Restless or unrefreshing sleep
- Muscle cramps or twitches
- A reliable afternoon energy crash
- Anxious or restless when I'm without my phone for a couple of hours
- Lonely or unseen even when I'm around people
- Drained more often than recharged after time with others

If several of these improve as you rework your top environments, that's your signal the architecture—not your willpower—was the problem.

A Note on the Evidence

The strength of the science behind these sections is not equal, and it's worth being honest about that:

- **Well-supported:** morning daylight and consistent sleep timing (Section 2); the harms of prolonged sitting and the value of daily movement (Section 3); the link between social connection and health (Section 7); the benefits of fermented foods and colorful, polyphenol-rich vegetables for the gut (parts of Section 5); the value of whole over ultra-processed food (parts of Sections 1 and 9).
- **More mixed or context-dependent:** Much of the Chemical section (Section 4)—heated plastics and worn nonstick are reasonable, low-cost things to avoid, but everyday exposures are debated and easy to overstate; and the Nutrients section (Section 9), where a true deficiency is worth correcting but routine supplementing "just in case" isn't automatically beneficial.

A high score flags an environment worth a closer look—not a verdict. For anything involving symptoms, medication, or supplements (especially Sections 4, 5, and 9), check with a clinician or get the relevant bloodwork before making big changes. I'm not a medical professional, and this tool can't see your individual situation.

Track your scores over time: This audit is a snapshot. The wellnessMAP app turns it into a living dashboard—re-take it as you redesign each environment, and watch which changes actually move your numbers.

Now go to the chapter that matches your highest score. You don't have to read this book in order. You have to read it in *your* order.

PART I
THE NINE ENVIRONMENTS

CHAPTER 1

The Food Environment

Let me ask you something.

It's nine o'clock at night. You already ate dinner—a good dinner, two hours ago. You're not hungry. And yet here you are, standing in front of the open cabinet, reaching for something. You're eating before you even decided to eat.

So what happened there?

Most people—and most doctors—will tell you that's a willpower problem. You're weak. You have no discipline. You just need to try harder.

That is *so* not true.

Here's what they don't tell you. The food around you is sending signals to your body twenty-four hours a day. Not just when you eat it. All the time. Whether you're hungry or not, whether you're paying attention or not—the food that's available to you, how engineered it is, how often it shows up, what form it comes in—all of that is information. And your metabolism is reading that information every single second.

Right now, almost all of it is wrong.

Now, the most common question I get is, "Dr. Berg, what should I eat?"

Wrong question.

The real question—the one almost nobody asks—is this: *what is my food environment doing to my body before I even make a choice?*

Because by the time you're standing at that cabinet at nine o'clock, the choice was already made for you. The environment made it.

This is not a willpower problem. It's an *architecture* problem. And once you see that, everything changes.

Your food is not calories. It's instruction.

What you might not know is that your body doesn't really see food as calories. It sees food as data. Every single meal is a message—it's answering questions your body has been asking for two and a half million years:

Is this a season of abundance, or scarcity? Are we safe, or are we stressed? What time of year is it? Are nutrients coming in, or are we running low? And how much work did it take to get this food?

For almost all of human history, those answers were accurate. Food was seasonal. Eating took effort—you had to hunt it, gather it, dig it out of the ground. Meals were events, not a constant drip all day long. And your body—boy, your body is smart—it built its entire operating system around those patterns.

Now here's the problem.

The modern food environment distorts every one of those signals. All of them. At the same time.

That's the villain in this chapter. Not sugar all by itself. Not fat all by itself. It's the environment—the whole engineered system you're swimming in—feeding your body false information from the second you wake up.

Let me show you exactly how. Then I'll show you how to fix it.

The Ways Your Food Environment Is Working Against You

Industrial food is the default now. Walk into any gas station, any airport, any office break room, any grocery store checkout line. What's sitting there? Packaged, shelf-stable, engineered food. Not food that evolved over thousands of years to match your biology—food that was designed by engineers to make you buy it again.

Here's the thing they don't tell you. That's not the exception anymore. That's the baseline. That's the default.

And when ultra-processed food is what's in front of you everywhere you go, it stops looking like a choice. It starts looking like "normal." And normal runs your behavior way faster than any piece of health information ever will.

Seed oils are hiding where you'd never expect. Restaurant cooking. Packaged snacks. Salad dressings. Sauces. Almost everything that's prepared for you commercially is cooked in industrial seed oils—soybean, corn, canola, sunflower.

Now, some people will tell you these oils are heart-healthy. That is so not true.

These oils are biologically foreign. Here's the number that matters: the ratio of omega-6 to omega-3 in the ancestral diet was about **4 to 1**. The modern Western diet runs **15 to 1, even 20 to 1**. That is not a little adjustment.

So, to make this simple: Your cells are built out of the fats you eat. The membrane around every single cell in your body is made from this stuff. Feed your body the wrong fat, and you're building every cell out of the wrong material. That's a membrane-level distortion, and it touches every cell you've got.

And you don't have to go looking for these oils. That's the trap. The environment delivers them to you automatically. Avoiding them is the thing that takes effort.

Liquid calories sneak right past your off switch. Juice. Smoothies. The big coffee drinks. Sports drinks. Soda.

Now here's something to think about. Ancestral humans had no liquid-calorie category. None. You drank water. Once in a while, milk. That's the entire list.

Liquid calories skip the chewing step—and chewing is not some little detail. Chewing turns on your satiety signals *before* the food even gets to your stomach. So liquid calories spike your insulin fast, they give you almost no fullness signal, and they pile on calories without your brain ever logging it as "a meal."

And the environment has built an entire liquid-calorie industry on top of that. Juice bars dress up as health food. A Frappuccino can hit 500 calories. Energy drinks bookend your whole workday. And not one of those flips the off switch.

Here's the clue, and you can test this on yourself today: Drink your calories, and an hour later you're hungry again.

Eat the same calories as *food* you have to chew, and you're not. That's your satiety system telling you which one your body actually counts.

This food was engineered to beat you. This one is worth stopping on.

Food scientists have a name for it: the "bliss point." Not that you needed to know the term, but it's the exact combination of sugar, fat, salt, and texture that maximizes what they call "hedonic response." In plain English? Eating when you're not hungry. Going past full. Thinking about the food after you've already stopped.

And here's what you have to understand—this is not an accident. It is optimized. The processed food industry is a **$1.2 trillion** business, and it pays researchers specifically to find the combinations that override your fullness and keep you eating.

So your willpower is not up against the craving. Your willpower is up against the entire research-and-development budget of multinational food corporations. The game is rigged—and it's rigged at the level of your environment, before you ever get to the kitchen.

Fix the environment. Take the engineering out. The cravings mostly disappear.

There's a trigger in every single room. Here's something that did not exist in any ancestral environment: food at every possible location, at every possible moment of the day.

Food at your desk. Food in the car. Candy at the pharmacy checkout. Snacks at the bank. Chips at the gas station. Cookies in the conference room.

Your metabolism evolved under what I'd call low opportunity—food took effort to get, and it showed up in specific situations. Hunting. Gathering. A meal. So when you felt hunger, it was *real* hunger. It was not a reaction to walking past a vending machine.

Modern life dropped a caloric trigger into every room you walk through. And the result is this: Your eating is now cue-driven, not hunger-driven. You eat because the food is there—not because your body asked for fuel. It's not a discipline problem. It's a trigger problem.

The clock took over for your body. Breakfast is mandatory. Lunch is at noon. Dinner is expected. Snacks are normal.

What you might not know is that none of those are biological requirements. They're cultural inventions. That whole idea that "breakfast is the most important meal of the day"? That was a marketing campaign—built by cereal companies back in the 1940s. It was never physiology. It was advertising.

So when the clock is driving your eating instead of your hunger, your body loses its main feedback signal. You eat before you need to. You keep eating past when you should've stopped. And your insulin goes up on schedule—whether your body needed it to or not.

And every time you raise insulin, you shut off fat-burning.

So eating on the clock, all day long, keeps insulin up, up, up—and keeps the fat locked in.

Modern food is too soft—and softness deletes a signal. It's pre-cut. Blended. A lot of it is basically liquid already.

Looks like convenience, right? It's actually a signal getting deleted.

Here's the mechanism. Chewing turns on what's called the cephalic phase of digestion. Not that you need the name—it just means a whole set of "get ready" responses that fire *before* the food ever reaches your stomach. Saliva. Stomach acid getting primed. Your fullness hormones—those start releasing at the jaw, not down in the gut.

Soft food collapses that whole signal. You eat faster, and you stop later. The feedback loop gets cut short. Texture is biological information—and the environment has quietly stripped it out.

Your metabolism was built for winter. Ancestral humans had fruit for a few months a year. Honey was rare. High-carb foods were genuinely seasonal. And your body had a smart response to that brief window of abundance: it stored fat—getting ready for the months when all of it disappeared.

That storage period is supposed to end. That's the whole point of it. The modern environment never lets it end.

Fruit is in the store year-round. Sugar is available every day. There is no metabolic winter anymore. So insulin never gets to rest. The store-fat signal never switches off.

And constant abundance signaling—in a body that was designed for the fluctuation—gives you chronically high insulin, fat storage that never reverses, and a metabolism that's lost its flexibility.

The whole food supply went lean-muscle-only. Go to any grocery store. What's for sale? Lean cuts. Skinless chicken. Boneless everything. Protein powder. It's muscle meat, muscle meat, muscle meat.

So what's missing? Organs. Bone marrow. Connective tissue. The collagen-rich cuts. Bone broth.

And this matters, because organ meats and connective tissue carry the nutrients muscle meat just doesn't have—real vitamin A, the actual retinol, not beta-carotene. Copper. Zinc. Vitamin K2. Glycine. Those are the cofactors your body runs your detox, your hormones, your collagen repair, and your immune system on.

The food supply quietly pulled nutrient density out of the default. Now you have to go out of your way to get what used to be standard in every single kitchen.

And it's not just that the organs disappeared—the muscle meat itself changed too. Conventional chicken, grain-finished beef, farmed fish—these aren't the same food your body evolved to run on. Pasture-raised and grass-fed animals carry a different fat profile, more omega-3s, more of the fat-soluble vitamins that live in the fat itself. Wild-caught fish carries what farmed fish doesn't. Whole eggs—yolk included—carry the choline and fat-soluble vitamins that egg whites alone don't. So "high-quality protein" isn't just about hitting a gram target. It's sourcing, it's the cut, and it's the form. Pasture-raised over conventional. Fattier cuts over lean. Wild-caught over farmed. Whole eggs over whites. None of that requires a special trip—most grocery stores carry the better option right next to the worse one. You're just choosing differently.

The Fasting Absence Principle

Now here's the most counterintuitive idea in this whole chapter. It's important enough that I want to say it as plainly as I can:

Fasting is not something you do. It's something that *happens*—when eating is inconvenient.

For most of human history, people didn't eat all the time, because food wasn't around all the time. The gap between meals wasn't a health strategy somebody came up with. It was just reality. And that gap—that stretch of absence—is exactly when your body does its most important repair work.

So what the heck happens in that gap? Fasting turns on autophagy. Not that you needed to know the word, but autophagy is just your body taking all the junk it doesn't need—damaged, broken-down cellular parts—and recycling it for fuel. It drops your insulin back down to baseline. It flips on the fat-burning pathways. It lets your gut rest and repair. It brings back your metabolic flexibility.

And here's the part you have to sit with: none of that can happen if food is always visible, always within reach, and always socially expected. The cleanup crew never gets to come in.

So if you want to create a fasting environment, you have to fix the food environment first. If the food is on your counter, you'll eat it. If it's offered to you every two hours, you'll take it. If eating is the default thing everybody does at every gathering, you'll go along with it.

Your food environment decides your fasting environment. There is no workaround.

Let me give you a real example. Me.

I am the poster child for this. If there are chips in the house, I will find them. Especially at night. Popcorn, chips, Doritos—that's my thing. And for years I told myself the same little lie: I'll just buy them every once in a while. Just sometimes. Right.

It does not work.

Here's what actually happens. The second I'm even a little stressed, or I'm tired because I didn't sleep well the night before, I go find those salty snacks. And I don't eat a little. I eat the whole bag.

Now, here's the part that proves the entire point of this chapter. I have *great* willpower with sweets. Sugar doesn't tempt me at all. So this was never a discipline problem—I've clearly got the discipline, I just spend it somewhere else. Salty is my downfall. And no amount of trying harder ever fixed it.

You know what finally fixed it? I made sure there were none of those foods within a ten-mile radius of me. You will not find chips in my house. Anywhere. I restructured my environment so there's so much friction between me and that food—so many barriers—that the late-night craving runs into a wall.

And I'll be honest with you—late at night, when I'm craving,

I'm still searching the house. The urge didn't disappear. But I tricked myself at the one moment that actually counts: the grocery store. I just don't buy it. And that one move has been hugely successful. No more bloating. Better sleep. Less belly fat. Huge.

So don't make the mistake I made for years. You don't out-willpower the bag. You just don't bring the bag home.

Here's the Real Target

Most nutrition advice is about what to put in your mouth. This chapter is about something underneath that—what your food environment is doing to you before you make any choice at all.

And here's the key. Everything I just walked you through—industrial food as the default, the seed oils, the liquid calories, the engineered reward, the trigger in every room, the clock running your meals, the soft food, the year-round sugar, the lean-muscle-only protein—these are not nine separate habits you fix one at a time.

They're a system. And they all work together.

The food is hyperpalatable. It's everywhere. It takes no effort. It comes with no texture. It's cut off from any seasonal signal. It's liquid as often as it's solid. And it's on a schedule that has nothing to do with your biology.

So you end up with a body getting constant abundance signals, constant insulin stimulation, and constant eating cues—inside a metabolic system that was built for fluctuation, for effort, and for absence.

Fix the architecture, and the signals change. Change the signals, and the biology follows. That's the whole game.

What to Actually Do

All right, let me get right to it. This isn't a thirty-step list—these are the high-leverage moves, the ones that change your environment first. Do these.

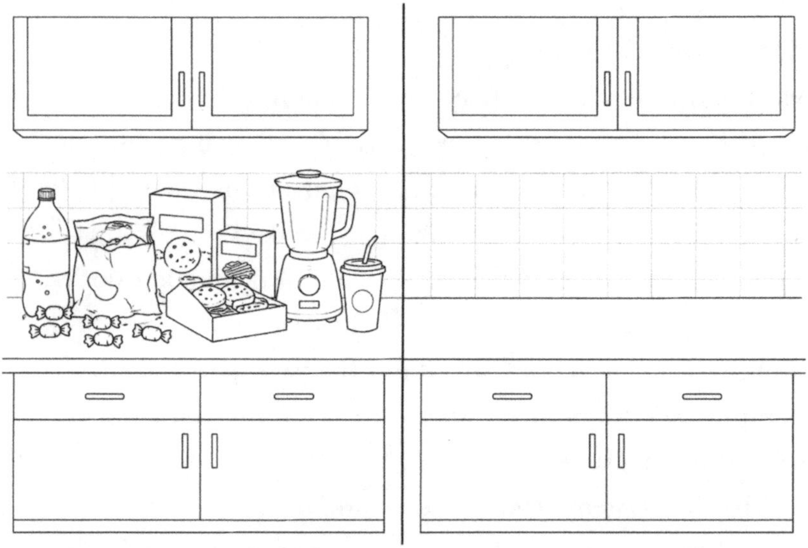

► START HERE

The one move that unlocks everything in Chapter 1:

Tonight, remove every snack food from your house. Not "put it in a harder-to-reach cabinet." Out of the house. This is the single move that closes the gap between knowing this chapter and living it. If it's not there, you can't eat it at 9:00 p.m. That's not willpower—that's architecture. Do this tonight. Everything else in this chapter compounds from here.

1. **Restructure what you see.** What's on your counter right now? Here's the rule—what you see is what you eat. And that cuts both ways. Most people hear it and think, great, I'll just leave a bowl of fruit out instead. Don't. If food is visible, you'll reach for it—not because you're hungry, but because it's there. Visible food is a cue, and a cue to eat between meals is the exact thing we're trying to remove. So clear the counter completely. Not mostly—bare. The engineered food goes out of the house entirely, because if it's there, I'll eat it. And don't leave the healthy stuff out as a consolation prize either—grazing on fruit all day still spikes insulin and still erases the gap your body needs. Same with the fridge and the pantry: Keep the grab-and-go food out of eye level, so opening the door isn't an invitation to snack. An empty counter gives your body no reason to eat until it's actually mealtime. That's the win.
2. **Build real meals with real gaps between them.** Two or three meals. Nothing in between. No snacks. Let your insulin fall between meals—that's the window where your body burns fat and does its repair work. This is not a diet. You're just restoring the pattern your body was built for.
3. **Give yourself a real overnight fast.** Stop eating three to four hours before bed, and don't eat again until you're genuinely hungry the next day. That's your fasting window—most people land somewhere between fourteen and eighteen hours without trying. Don't chase

a number. Let the gap happen, the way it would have happened for most of human history. This is where the repair work in the section above actually takes place.

4. **Cut the liquid calories.** Water. Coffee or tea with nothing caloric in it. This one change pulls out a massive source of insulin stimulation, and you won't even feel deprived—because liquid calories never made you full in the first place.
5. **Put the chewing back.** Pick foods you actually have to chew. Real meat, not processed. Raw vegetables, not preblended. Hard cheese, not the spreadable stuff. Whole nuts, not the nut butter. The chewing is doing metabolic work for you.
6. **Eat with the seasons.** Not perfectly—just pull the fruit back toward summer, ease off the starchy stuff in winter, and stop treating sugar like a daily year-round staple. That gives your insulin system the rest it was designed to get.
7. **Upgrade your protein, not just your portion.** Pasture-raised over conventional. Fattier cuts over lean. Wild-caught over farmed. Whole eggs over whites. This one swap fixes most of what the lean-muscle-only food supply stripped out—and it's the move to make before you're ready for organ meats.
8. **Add organ meat once a week.** If you want to maximize nutrient density, beef liver once a week is the highest-return food in this chapter. Start small.

The Bottom Line

Your food environment is engineered against you right now. And I don't mean that as a figure of speech—it was literally designed that way, by people who are paid specifically to maximize how much you consume.

So the solution was never better willpower. The solution is a different environment.

Change what's available, what's visible, what's within reach, what's expected. Change the form your food takes. Change the timing. Change the frequency.

And the biology takes care of the rest.

And remember, the food environment never acts alone. What you put on your plate is also feeding—or starving—the microbiome you'll meet in Chapter 5, and the most processed foods tend to carry the heaviest chemical load too (Chapter 4). Fix this one environment and you've already started moving both of those.

Now—there's a second system that has to be working before any of this fully lands, and it's the one most people never even think about. Your timing system. Your body cannot repair what the food environment damaged if it doesn't know what time it is. And right now, dim days and bright nights are doing more metabolic damage to you than almost anything on your plate.

That's Chapter 2—Light and Sleep. I'll see you there.

CHAPTER 2

Light and Sleep

Most people think sleep is a habit problem.

Go to bed earlier. Put your phone down. Try melatonin. Cut the caffeine. And if none of that works—well, maybe you just have bad sleep. Some people do, right?

That is *so* not true.

Sleep isn't a habit problem. It's a timing problem. Your body shuts down on a cue—the one that tells it it's finally safe—and that cue isn't coming from a supplement or a bedtime routine. It's coming from light.

Specifically, the light you're not getting during the day, and the light you're getting too much of at night.

Our biology evolved around the circadian light and dark daily cycle.

Now, the problem with treating this as a habit is that it sends you after the wrong target. You optimize the bedroom, you buy a sleep tracker, you try magnesium—and it helps a little, but nothing fully works. Because you're working far down the road of the actual problem. The real issue is that your biological clock doesn't know what time it is. And the reason it doesn't know what time it is, is that your light environment has erased the clock.

Let me explain what I mean.

Your body doesn't know time from clocks. It knows time from light. There's a tiny structure in your brain called the suprachiasmatic nucleus—the SCN. Not that you needed to know the name of it, but this is your master clock.

Every cell in your body runs its own little internal timer, and the SCN is the thing that keeps all of them synchronized. Hormones, metabolism, immune function, digestion, repair—all of it runs on a twenty-four-hour cycle, and all of it takes its timing instructions from that one clock.

Now here's what's interesting. The SCN doesn't take its instructions from your calendar or your alarm. It takes them from light and darkness. But more specifically, from light hitting specialized cells in the back of your retina. Those cells carry a photopigment—you don't need the name—but it's especially sensitive to blue-wavelength light. Daylight. The kind of light the sun puts out in the morning.

When that light hits those cells, it fires a message up to the SCN that says: it's daytime, wake up. Start the clock. Release cortisol. Raise body temperature. Activate.

When that signal stops—when it gets dark—the clock shifts the other way. Melatonin starts rising. Body temperature drops. The body starts moving toward sleep, toward repair, toward shutdown.

That's the system. It's been running for two hundred thousand years, and it works perfectly—when the light environment is right.

The modern light environment is not right. And that's the whole problem.

The most damaging light pattern is dim days and bright nights. And this is the thing almost nobody gets right.

The most damaging light environment isn't staying up too late once in a while. It isn't the odd screen before bed. Those are minor disruptions—your body can handle them. The real damage is the combination: dim days, bright nights.

Think about what modern indoor life actually looks like. You wake up, you're inside. You work inside, under overhead lighting—maybe 200 to 500 lux, which sounds bright until you find out that outdoor daylight runs 10,000 to 100,000 lux (lux being simply how bright a light is as it lands on a surface).

You drive home inside a car. You cook and eat and spend your whole evening inside—and now the lights are on, the screens are on, and you're getting 300 to 1,000 lux straight into your retina until eleven o'clock at night.

So here's what your biology is receiving: a weak, ambiguous day signal—followed immediately by a strong, unmistakable bright signal at night.

From the perspective of your master clock, that's not a schedule. That's noise. There's no strong start signal in the morning, and no strong stop signal at night. The clock can't anchor. It drops into what I think of as a biological gray zone—not fully awake, not fully asleep, not fully anything. Partial-day mode, all the time.

And what does that feel like? You probably already know. You sleep eight hours and wake up exhausted. You've got a low-grade anxiety with no clear cause. You're wired at midnight and foggy at ten in the morning. Fat loss stalls even when the diet is right. You crash every single afternoon.

That's not a sleep problem. That's a clock erasure. Your clock has lost the light/dark contrast it needs to work.

Darkness doesn't make you sleep. It gives your body the all-clear. This is the insight that changes everything.

Here's the thing. Your body doesn't sleep by force. It sleeps on a signal—and the signal it's waiting for is safety.

Darkness doesn't force your body to sleep. What darkness does is remove the signal that's been telling your body it's not safe to shut down. When the light disappears—real darkness, not "dark enough"—your brain reads that as safety. It's safe to be vulnerable now and relax. It's safe to repair. It's safe to shut the defenses off and do maintenance.

Without that signal, your body won't fully commit to deep sleep. It stays in a lighter, more alert state. Not because you're not tired—you're exhausted. It's because the nervous system never got the all-clear. The signal never came.

Now, this is exactly why melatonin supplements don't work for most people. You're adding the hormone after the fact while the light signal is still telling your brain it's two in the afternoon. You can't supplement your way around a bad environment. I've seen this so many times in practice—people taking five to ten milligrams of melatonin and still lying there wide awake. The dose was never the problem. The environment is the problem.

Fix the environment, and the signal comes through on its own.

Here's the hormone cascade. Once you see it, the whole picture makes sense.

Morning light hits the retina, the SCN fires, and cortisol peaks. And that's healthy—your morning cortisol is supposed to be high. It's what wakes you up, gives you mental clarity, gets glucose moving. The problem is, if you're not getting bright morning light, that cortisol peak gets blunted. You wake up flat. And now you need three cups of coffee just to fake what your body should be doing on its own.

Through the day, cortisol is supposed to slide down gradually. By evening—if the light has been dimming naturally—cortisol is low, melatonin is rising, and your core temperature is dropping. That drop in temperature is actually one of the key triggers for sleep. Your body uses it as a shutdown signal.

Bright light at night disrupts every single step of that cascade. It suppresses melatonin—and here's what most people don't realize: ordinary household lighting is plenty to do it. You don't have to be staring at a screen. The overhead LEDs in your kitchen. The bathroom light when you get up at 2:00 a.m. The hallway light glowing through the bedroom door. That's enough. Visual brightness is not the same thing as circadian safety.

And what about growth hormone? Growth hormone surges in the first few hours of deep sleep—specifically in slow-wave sleep. That's your main tissue-repair window. Muscle, bone, collagen, immune cells. If you're not getting deep sleep, because the light environment suppressed your melatonin and kept cortisol elevated into the evening, that growth hormone surge gets cut short—or lost completely. You're not repairing properly. Repair happens mostly during sleep—but only if that sleep is actually deep.

I remember in basic training in the army, they kept us up for several days in a row and added physical exercise and stress from the drill sergeant. No repair, high sustained cortisol stress and wicked blood sugar problems on top of it. Talk about the opposite of "safety" signals.

The daytime problem is actually bigger than the nighttime problem. Some people hear all this and fixate on the night side. Screens off. Blue-light glasses. Blackout curtains.

Those things matter—but they're only half the equation. Here's the part that took me a while to fully appreciate: Night light is most damaging when the day was too dim.

Think about it. Before electricity, people had campfire light, candlelight, firelight every single night. Orange, warm, fairly bright—and right up close to the eye. And it didn't wreck their sleep. Why not? Because the day had been spent in full outdoor light: 10,000 to 100,000 lux. The clock had been anchored so hard in the morning that it could tolerate an imperfect evening signal.

The contrast was enormous. Blazing bright days. Relatively dark nights with a little warm firelight. And that contrast is exactly what the clock was built for.

What we've done with modern indoor life is collapse that contrast in both directions at once.

Here's why firelight never disrupted ancestral sleep—and why modern LEDs do. It comes down to one specific wavelength.

Your master clock isn't sensitive to all light equally. The cells in your retina that set your circadian timing respond most powerfully to short-wavelength blue light—around 480 nanometers. That's the wavelength the morning sky is full of. It's the wake-up signal.

Firelight, candlelight, and the old incandescent bulbs have almost none of it. Their light is warm—orange and red spectrum—sitting well above 600 nanometers. So your ancestors could sit around a fire for hours after dark and their master clock barely registered it. The signal wasn't there.

Modern LEDs are different. They're engineered for efficiency, and they're loaded with blue-spectrum output—the exact wavelength that tells your brain it's midday. Ordinary household LED lighting at night can suppress melatonin by up to 50 percent. Not the extreme brightness—just the spectrum. Your kitchen overhead light is doing this to you every evening.

So the real reason firelight was safe isn't magic—it's physics. The wavelength that resets your clock wasn't in it. The wavelength in your LED ceiling fixture is. That's the swap your biology never agreed to, and it's happening in every room of your house, every night.

So if you want to fix your sleep environment, start with the day. Get outside within thirty to sixty minutes of waking up. No sunglasses at first—let your retina take in the full-spectrum signal. Even on a cloudy day, outdoor light runs 1,000 to 10,000 lux, which is dramatically more than anything you get indoors. Ten minutes is the minimum. Twenty to forty-five minutes is better. This one habit—morning outdoor light—is the single most powerful circadian intervention there is. It sets the clock for the entire day downstream.

Now here's where Chapter 1 and Chapter 2 connect. And this one surprised me when I first really understood it.

Your food timing directly affects your sleep architecture.

When you eat late—within two to three hours of bed—a few things happen. Blood sugar rises. Insulin rises. Body temperature stays up, because digestion is metabolically active. And then, usually between two and four in the morning, your blood sugar drops. Your body reads that drop as a low-fuel emergency, and it releases adrenaline to push the glucose back up.

For many people, that adrenaline spike is what causes the 3:00 a.m. wakeup that seems to come from nowhere.

It's not anxiety. It's not insomnia. It's a blood sugar event—one your environment triggered, by the timing of your last meal. So close the kitchen three to four hours before bed. Eat protein and fat at dinner instead of heavy carbohydrates. Let your blood sugar stabilize before sleep. For most people, those 3:00 a.m. wakeups resolve within a week or two.

Now combine that with what we covered in Chapter 1—eating in a real window, with real gaps, not grazing until 10:00 p.m. You're not just fixing the food environment. You're protecting the sleep environment at the same time. These systems talk to each other. Get the food timing right, and the sleep tightens up. Get the light right, and the next day's cravings drop—because poor sleep raises ghrelin, your hunger hormone, and lowers leptin, your satiety hormone. Bad sleep makes you hungry. Better sleep makes the whole food environment easier to manage.

They're not separate chapters. They're the same system.

The Architecture That Actually Works

Let me tell you how I learned this one. The hard way, of course.

My sleep problems started back in basic training. I had a drill sergeant who woke me up—rudely, at 4:00 a.m. every single morning. And that reprogrammed my clock. It set a new time, and my body held on to it years after.

But here's where I made it worse. Years later, I started bragging about how early I got up—how I was getting a head start on everybody else. Boy, that was stupid. Because what I was *actually* doing was running on five and a half hours of sleep. For years.

And I had no idea what it was costing me. The short sleep, stacked on top of sitting at a computer twelve-plus hours a day—it was wrecking me. Tired all the time. Brain fog. My whole body felt inflamed.

It didn't turn around until I stumbled onto the power of morning sunlight. That was the piece I'd been missing. The contrast. Thirty minutes of bright sunlight in the morning, complete darkness at night, and dimming my lights three hours before bed. That's when everything changed. Now I sleep eight-plus hours, and my brain and my body have healed because of it.

Don't make the mistakes I made. The fix wasn't complicated. It was environmental.

Most people try to improve their sleep by adding things. A supplement. A routine. A device. The real move is removing what's blocking it.

So here's the architecture that actually changes the environment:

► START HERE

The one move that unlocks everything in Chapter 2:
Tomorrow morning, go outside within thirty minutes of waking. No sunglasses. Ten minutes minimum. Don't check your phone first. Just go out and stand in the light. This single habit—done before anything else—sets your cortisol peak, anchors your circadian clock, and pulls every other sleep improvement downstream. You can do everything else in this chapter imperfectly and this one move will still carry most of the benefit. Start here.

1. **Fix the morning first.** Outside within thirty to sixty minutes of waking. No sunglasses for that first exposure. Ten minutes minimum, twenty to forty-five is better. Do it before anything else—before coffee if you can. This is the highest-ROI single habit in this entire chapter, and it costs nothing.
2. **Same wake time every day.** This one is non-negotiable. The clock stabilizes off your wake time, not your bedtime—even if you went to bed late, even on weekends. Allow yourself thirty minutes of variance, not two hours. Two hours of weekend drift and you've handed yourself Monday jet lag, every single week.

3. **Overhead lights off at sunset.** Lamps only. Warm-spectrum bulbs. This is harder than it sounds, because it means changing the default in every room of the house. But overhead LED lighting at night is one of the primary circadian disruptors in the modern home. Dimmer switches help. Pre-set it so you're not making the decision every night—if you have to choose in the moment, the friction is too high.
4. **Make the bedroom a zero-light zone.** Not dim. Dark. Blackout curtains. Every LED covered or removed—the standby light on the TV, the charging indicator on the power strip, the glow of a clock. Sounds excessive, until you understand that your retina is detecting light even when your eyes are closed. Any light signal at night is biological information being received. Darkness is an active signal—it's not the absence of something, it's the presence of the safety instruction your nervous system needs.
5. **Phone out of the bedroom.** This is both a light issue and a nervous-system issue. The physical act of reaching for the phone during a night waking—even just to check the time—triggers alertness, blue light, and cortisol. Remove the option entirely. Use an analog alarm clock. The phone charges in another room. This one change, all by itself, improves sleep for most people within a week.
6. **Kitchen closed three to four hours before bed.** Brush your teeth. Turn the kitchen lights off. Take late eating off the table—literally. This protects the blood sugar stability that protects your sleep, like we just covered.

7. **Screens end before biological night.** Two to three hours before sleep is ideal. And "night mode" is not a solution—it cuts the blue light somewhat, but melanopsin responds to overall light intensity as much as spectrum. Night mode just gives you an excuse to keep staring at a bright screen. That is not the same as putting it away.

Redesign Your Light Environment

This is the part you actually control. You can't change the sun, but you can change almost everything about the light you live in.

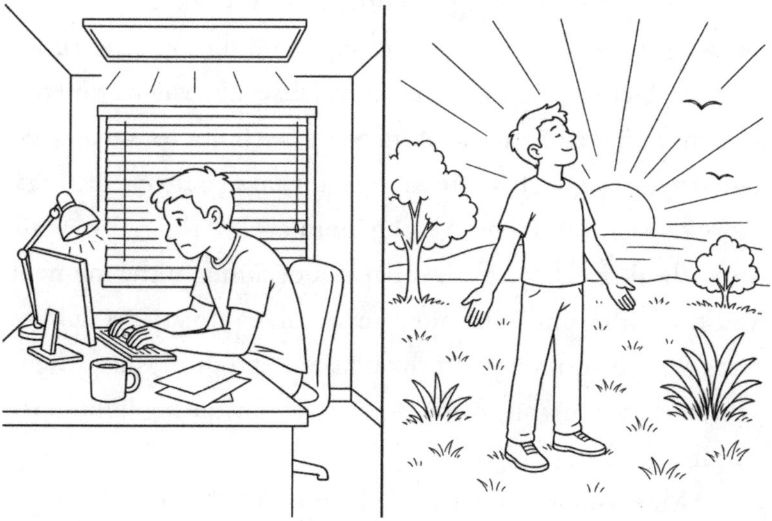

All right, here's where it gets real. Same as the kitchen—put the book down and actually walk through your house. Don't save it for tomorrow, don't wait for the weekend. Do it now, while it's in front of you. We're going to do three passes: set the morning, kill the bright nights, black out the bedroom. That's the whole redesign.

Pass one—set the morning. This is the highest-leverage thing in the whole chapter, so we build the environment to make it automatic. Walk to the door you'll actually go out of tomorrow morning, and set the path now. Shoes by that door. A chair on the porch, the balcony, the back step—wherever you'll really stand in the light. If you drink coffee, decide right now you'll drink it outside. The goal is zero decisions at 7:00 a.m.—you just walk out into the light because everything's already in place. Don't rely on remembering. Rely on the setup.

Pass two—kill the bright nights. Now walk the house at night-light level. Every overhead light you flip on after sunset is the problem—so go find the lamps instead. One warm lamp in each room you actually sit in. Swap the bulbs to warm-spectrum if you've got them; if you don't, that's your one purchase out of this entire chapter. Set the dimmers low right now, while you're thinking about it, so you're not deciding in the moment. And the bathroom—the one you stumble into at 2:00 a.m.—that's the worst offender in the house. Put a dim, warm night-light in there tonight, so you never reach for the big light in the middle of the night again.

Pass three—black out the bedroom. Walk into where you sleep and hunt for light. Every little glowing dot—the standby light on the TV, the charger indicator, the cable box, the face of the clock. Cover them. Tape, a sticker, unplug it, turn it to the wall—I don't care how, just kill every point of light in the room. Curtains that actually block the streetlight, not the ones that sort of help. And the phone charges in another room starting tonight—get an analog alarm clock if that's the one thing stopping you. Your retina reads light even with your eyes closed, so the bar here isn't "dim enough." It's dark.

That's it. When you're done, your evenings should look different than they did ten minutes ago—lower, warmer, softer—and your bedroom should be a cave. If nothing in your house actually changed, you didn't redesign your environment—you just read about it. Go back and do the three passes for real. That's the difference between knowing this chapter and sleeping on it.

The Fourteen-Day Reset

If your sleep is significantly broken right now, here's the fastest path to resetting the clock.

Fourteen days. Enforce five things—only these five:

1. Fixed wake time—same every day, no exceptions.
2. Morning outdoor light within thirty minutes of waking.
3. Phone out of the bedroom.
4. Kitchen closed three to four hours before bed.
5. Darkness after sunset—lamps only, no overhead lights.

That's it. Don't add supplements. Don't optimize further. Just those five, enforced hard, for fourteen days.

Most people see dramatic improvement in seven to ten days. Not because they found some new technique—because they removed what was blocking sleep from happening. Your body already knows how to sleep. You just have to stop interfering with it.

The Bottom Line

Light is not ambiance. Light is instruction.

Your body uses it to know what time it is—when to be awake, when to shut down, when to repair. When the light environment gives accurate information—bright days, dark nights, consistent timing—the system runs exactly as designed. Sleep is deep. Hormones are timed. Repair happens. Metabolism works.

The modern light environment gives inaccurate information. Dim days that fail to anchor the clock. Bright nights that prevent shutdown. The result isn't a sleep disorder. It's a timing disorder. And the fix isn't a pill. It's a different environment.

Fix the day first. Then fix the night. The body takes care of the rest.

Light and sleep sit upstream of nearly everything else in this book. Get this environment right and you'll feel it in your food cravings (Chapter 1), your stress, and your focus (Chapter 6)—often before you deliberately change anything else. If you fix only one environment in this whole book, make it this one.

Next chapter: Movement. Not exercise—movement. There's a difference, and it matters more than most people realize. Your body was built for low-level, constant movement all day long—not one hour at the gym followed by eight hours stuck in a chair. We'll get into why sedentary environments do metabolic damage that exercise can't fully undo—and exactly what to change in your space to fix it.

CHAPTER 3

Movement, Work, and the Stress Drain

I want to tell you about two of my neighbors.

They're older than me. They help out on my farm once in a while—pulling the tractor out of the mud, running heavy equipment, digging out a pond. Hard, physical, outdoor work. The kind that takes most of the day.

Here's what they eat: pure junk food. One of them smokes. The other chews tobacco. If I described their diet and their lifestyle to any doctor in the country, I'd get the same answer every time—these men should be in serious trouble. Heart disease. Metabolic syndrome. Cancer risk. The standard projections.

Except they're not in trouble. They're older than me, and they're out there in the sun doing things I'd struggle to keep up with.

Now, I'm not telling you this because junk food is fine or tobacco doesn't matter—neither of those is true. I'm telling you this because these two men are demonstrating something I've gotten more and more convinced of over the years: The power of physical movement—real movement, outdoors, in the sun—is a bigger contributor to your health than most of us have ever been willing to admit.

Think about what their days look like. They're outside from morning to late afternoon. Constant low-level movement, interrupted by bursts of heavy exertion. Natural light all day long. They're never sitting at a desk. And they're using their bodies for something with a purpose—a real outcome, not reps on a machine.

Their food environment is genuinely terrible. And they're doing just fine.

Now think about what would happen if they also ate well.

That's what this chapter is about. But the reason they're thriving isn't magic—it comes down to something the modern health conversation almost never talks about.

Here's the thing nobody says out loud about the modern health crisis. We didn't just change what we eat. We also stopped moving.

Not stopped exercising—stopped moving. There's a difference, and it matters.

For almost all of human history, movement was inseparable from daily life. You didn't go to the gym and then sit for ten hours. Movement was how you got food, built shelter, moved yourself around, managed land, raised animals. It was woven into every hour. Your body got loaded and unloaded all day long—carrying, lifting, walking, digging, crouching, climbing.

And here's what almost nobody talks about. Physical work was also your primary way of draining stress.

When something threatened you—a predator, a conflict, a crisis—your body flooded with adrenaline and cortisol. Blood glucose spiked. Muscles tensed. Heart rate jumped. The whole stress response was preparing you to move.

And then you moved. You ran, you fought, you worked, you walked home. The physical exertion burned through the stress hormones. Cortisol dropped. Adrenaline cleared. The nervous system came back down.

That's the complete stress cycle. Activation, then physical discharge, then recovery.

What does the modern stress cycle look like? You get an email that makes your blood pressure spike. Cortisol floods your system. Blood glucose rises. Your body is fully prepared to physically respond.

And then you sit there. You type a reply. You sit some more.

Those stress hormones that got released to fuel movement have nowhere to go. They don't get metabolized. They stay up. Cortisol stays high into the evening. Inflammation builds. Sleep suffers. And tomorrow it happens again.

Walking was the drain valve. We removed the drain valve. Then we wondered why stress became chronic.

Now, this next part is the finding that changed how I think about the whole movement question. And I want to be clear about it, because it runs counter to what most people believe.

An hour at the gym does not cancel eight hours of sitting.

I know that sounds wrong. It sounds like the math should work—you exercised, you burned the calories, you moved. But the research is consistent on this: Prolonged sitting produces metabolic effects that are largely independent of whether you exercised earlier that day. Lipoprotein lipase—an enzyme that's critical for fat metabolism, not that you needed the name—drops dramatically within hours of continuous sitting. Insulin sensitivity degrades. Circulation to the lower body slows way down.

These are not effects a morning workout fully reverses. They're effects of the architecture—of a body designed for constant low-level movement being held still for most of its waking hours.

My neighbors never sit for eight hours. They couldn't if they tried. Their work builds the movement in. There's no equivalent in a modern office.

So the question isn't just "Are you exercising?" The real question is: "What does your movement environment look like for the other twenty-three hours?"

Let me describe a typical modern office to you, from a biological standpoint.

You sit for one to three hours. You walk to a meeting room—maybe 50 to 200 steps. You sit for another hour. You walk to the kitchen—another 50 steps. You sit until 5:00 p.m., get in your car, sit for 30 to 60 minutes, and arrive home. Total steps for the day: maybe 2,000. Total time in natural light: maybe twenty minutes. Total time in genuine physical movement: under ten minutes of actual walking, none of it continuous.

That's not an exaggeration. That's a normal day for millions of people.

Now here's what that environment is doing to your body

during those eight hours of sitting. Spinal loading shifts off the muscles—where it belongs—and onto the passive structures: the discs, the ligaments, the facet joints. Your hip flexors adaptively shorten. Your glutes go neurologically quiet—they actually stop firing correctly, because they haven't needed to. The upper back rounds. The head drifts forward. And boy, forward head posture loads your neck with tens of pounds of extra force—all because the screen is at the wrong height. We'll get into exactly what that does, and the numbers behind it, in Chapter 8.

Meanwhile, circulation slows. Lymph—which has no pump of its own, and depends entirely on muscle movement to get anywhere—stagnates. The diaphragm gets compressed. Breathing goes shallow. Oxygen delivery drops. Carbon dioxide stays elevated in the tissues.

None of this is dramatic enough to feel like a crisis in the moment. But it accumulates, daily, for years—and it produces a body that's structurally adapted to sitting. Which means structurally unadapted to everything else.

And here's the part people get wrong: The fix is not a standing desk. Standing still for eight hours is not better than sitting still for eight hours. The fix is movement variety—changing positions often, building in real movement breaks, and redesigning the work environment so that staying stationary for more than forty-five minutes takes effort.

So here's what actually works at a desk. Set yourself a movement alarm—not a suggestion, an alarm—every forty-five to sixty minutes, and when it goes off, you stand up and move for five minutes. Walk to the end of the building and back. That's not a productivity interruption. It's the thing that keeps you cognitively functional for the next hour, because circulation is oxygen delivery, and oxygen delivery is cognitive performance. Take any call that doesn't need a screen on your feet—outside if you can. Build friction into sitting: put the printer somewhere inconvenient, take the stairs, park farther away. Don't make movement a decision—make the inconvenient option the default. My neighbors don't decide to move; their environment requires it.

And here's something almost nobody thinks about: At that screen, it's not only your body that freezes—it's also your eyes, your neck, and your whole posture, locked in one fixed position for hours. That's a different kind of damage than sitting, and movement alone won't fully undo it. The desk earns its own chapter for exactly that reason—we'll get into the eyes, the screen light, the posture, and the specific fixes in Chapter 8.

And every hour you stay stationary, that cortisol has nowhere to go.

Now, I want to say something about walking specifically—because modern fitness culture dismisses it as "not real exercise," and that is completely backward.

Walking is the most fundamental physical output the human body has. It's continuous, rhythmic, low-impact, bilateral. It uses the entire kinetic chain. It promotes lymphatic flow, stimulates the vagus nerve, lowers cortisol, improves insulin sensitivity—and when you do it outside, it delivers the light signal, the fresh air, and the contact with nature your nervous system was built to receive, all at the same time.

A twenty- to thirty-minute walk after dinner blunts your post-meal blood sugar spike significantly—and I don't mean that as a figure of speech. The research on post-meal walking is remarkably consistent. The glucose spike gets blunted, the insulin response is reduced, and the food you just ate is far less likely to get stored as fat.

Walking after meals. Walking during phone calls. Walking in the morning for the light signal. Walking when you're stressed. Walking is not the consolation prize for people who can't do "real" exercise. It's the baseline movement your body expects every single day—and most people aren't getting it.

That twenty-minute walk after dinner isn't just blood sugar management. It's the drain valve your ancestors pulled every single day.

All this talk about walking and daily movement sometimes leads people to think they don't need real exercise.

They do.

Your body wasn't only designed for constant low-level movement. It was also designed for occasional high-intensity exertion. Sprinting from a predator. Carrying a heavy animal back to camp. A sustained burst of effort at maximum or near-maximum output—followed by rest and recovery.

That pattern—brief, intense effort, then recovery—is exactly what high-intensity interval training is mimicking. And it mimics it fairly well.

Here's what brief, intense exercise does that moderate steady cardio largely doesn't: It triggers a significant growth hormone surge—your repair-and-regeneration signal. It creates an acute metabolic stress that drives mitochondrial adaptation—your cells build more energy-generating machinery to handle the demand. It improves insulin sensitivity in a way that persists for twenty-four to forty-eight hours. It raises your metabolic rate after the workout's over—the body keeps burning at an elevated rate for hours after you stop. And it takes twenty minutes.

Twenty minutes of genuine high-intensity interval training—real intensity, not a moderate jog with a HIIT label slapped on it—produces metabolic adaptations that forty-five minutes of steady-state cardio doesn't reliably produce.

The ancestral version of this wasn't voluntary. You sprinted because something was chasing you. The effort was total and the duration was short. You didn't warm up first. You didn't have a recovery drink afterward.

The modern version— thirty to forty seconds of maximum effort, ninety seconds of recovery, repeated six to eight times—captures the core stimulus without needing a predator. Two to three sessions a week is enough. More is not better, and may be worse—because the recovery between sessions is where the adaptation actually happens.

The sprint wasn't optional for them. For us, it has to be.

And the best version of that all-out effort isn't in a gym at all.

Here's something the fitness industry will never tell you: Purposeful physical work is better exercise than most gym programs.

When you're building something, fixing something, digging, hauling, carrying, farming, your body is engaged in ways isolated resistance training doesn't replicate. You're using the full kinetic chain, not individual muscle groups. You're moving in three-dimensional space, not along a fixed machine path. You're doing it for a purpose, with a visible outcome. And you're usually doing it outside.

My neighbors are the proof. They're not following a training program. They're doing work. And that work is keeping them alive and functional in a way no structured gym program—the kind they'd never follow anyway—ever could.

Now, I'm not telling you to skip the gym. I'm telling you this: If you've got a choice between an hour at the gym and two hours of physical work outdoors—building, fixing, gardening, farming, whatever it is—the second option is not the inferior one. It might be the better one.

Purpose-driven effort also engages your nervous system differently. When you're lifting because the task requires it—not because a program says three sets of ten—the movement is integrated. Your brain is coordinating, not running a script. And that coordination has its own benefits—balance, proprioception, spatial awareness—that machine-based exercise mostly bypasses.

There's one more thing my neighbors are getting that the desk worker isn't—and it's the one nobody talks about. Oxygen.

Modern sedentary environments produce a chronic, mild hypoxia—not enough to feel like you're suffocating, but enough to affect your mitochondrial function, your mental clarity, your cellular energy production. Indoor air is typically worse than outdoor air. Shallow, sitting-posture breathing cuts your tidal volume. And a sedentary life means you never demand a deep oxygen exchange.

Physical exertion—especially outside—forces your respiratory system to work fully. Deep breathing activates the parasympathetic nervous system. Oxygen delivery to your brain goes up. Carbon dioxide, which is a vasodilator, gets regulated correctly. The whole system gets flushed out.

This is part of why those two men—even with the poor diet, even with the tobacco—carry a metabolic buffer that desk workers don't have. The oxygen environment, the light environment, and the movement environment are all working correctly at the same time. It's not one thing. It's the combination.

What to Actually Do

► START HERE

The one move that unlocks everything in Chapter 3:

Set a repeating alarm on your phone for every fifty minutes during your workday. Label it: MOVE. When it goes off, stand up and walk—to the end of the building, around the block, up the stairs, anywhere. Five minutes. Do not stretch at your desk. Move through space. This one change—enforced by your phone, not your memory—breaks the metabolic damage of prolonged sitting more effectively than any exercise session added at the end of the day. Start here.

1. **Anchor the after-meal walk to something already in the room.** Even ten minutes is the highest-return single habit in this chapter—blood sugar, digestion, cortisol, lymphatic flow all improve. So don't leave it to memory. Put your shoes by the door you actually leave from, the leash on the hook, and tie the walk to a cue that already happens every day—dishes done, kettle on, dog waiting at the door. The walk should be triggered by your kitchen, not by your willpower.
2. **Make staying still take effort.** Keep the movement alarm—every forty-five to sixty minutes, five minutes of real movement through space, not stretching at your desk. But build the room to back it up: Move your charger, your water, the trash can, and the printer far enough from your seat that getting up is forced rather than chosen.
3. **Leave the gear out so the session has no setup.** Two to three HIIT sessions a week—real intensity, thirty to forty seconds of maximum effort, ninety seconds of recovery, six to eight rounds. Twenty minutes total. What kills it isn't the effort, it's the friction beforehand. Lay the gear out the night before, put the bike or the rope where you trip over it, pick something that needs zero assembly. Take the steps out from between you and the work.
4. **Default your calls to audio.** Every call that doesn't need a screen should happen on your feet, outside if you can. Set it up so the walking version is the easy one—headset

on the hook by the door, camera off by default—so you don't have to decide to walk. You'd have to decide not to.

5. **Install a standing physical obligation.** A garden that has to be tended, a woodpile, a workshop, animals, a project with a deadline—purposeful physical work with a visible outcome. Don't schedule it like a gym session you can skip. Set it up as something that pulls the movement out of you whether you feel like it or not. That's what my neighbors have. The work decides; they just show up.
6. **Move a daily trigger outdoors.** The light, the air, the uneven ground, the change of scenery add a signal layer indoor movement just doesn't. So put something you need every day—the morning coffee, the morning light, the route to anything—where you have to step outside to reach it. Make outdoors the path, not the detour.

Redesign Your Movement Environment

Before you try to do any of that, walk through the three places your day actually happens and change them once—so movement is the default and sitting still is the thing that takes effort. This is the same move as clearing the kitchen. You're not promising to behave better. You're rebuilding the room so the right thing happens on its own.

1. **Your desk.** Pull everything you reach for off the desk—charger, water, snacks, trash can, printer—and put it far enough away that you have to stand to get it. Raise the

monitor to eye level; add a stand if you're on a laptop. The goal is a workstation that interrupts you, not one that lets you fossilize in place for three hours.

2. **Your home.** Stage the friction-free version of every movement you want. Walking shoes by the door you actually use. Headset on the hook for calls. The after-dinner walk tied to a cue that already happens. Workout gear left out, not packed away. If a movement needs setup, you won't do it. If it's already laid out, you will.
3. **Your daily path.** Look at the route your body takes through an ordinary day and add the steps back in on purpose. Park at the far end. Make the stairs the easy choice and the elevator the slow one. Put the thing you fetch most often upstairs or outside. And install one standing physical obligation—a garden, a project, animals—that drags you out of the chair on its own schedule.

None of this is willpower. You're just taking away the chair's monopoly on your day.

The Bottom Line

Your body was designed to move constantly, work hard occasionally, and be outside doing both.

The modern environment removed all three at once—and replaced them with a chair, a screen, and a one-hour gym session three times a week that's supposed to make up for the other 165 hours.

It can't. The math doesn't work, and the biology doesn't work.

My neighbors—with their terrible diet, their tobacco, their junk food—are proof of what movement and sun can do even when everything else is wrong. Now imagine what they'd do if everything else were right.

Fix the movement environment. Build real gaps into the desk day. Walk with purpose. Sprint once in a while. Work with your body when you can. Get outside.

The body knows what to do. It just needs an environment that asks it to.

Movement doesn't stay in its own lane either. The same sitting that stalls your metabolism is built into the workspace you'll redesign in Chapter 8—and when your movement happens outdoors, it's doing double duty as your light environment from Chapter 2.

Next chapter: The Chemical Environment. Your home and your workplace are saturated with compounds your biology has never encountered before—in your cleaning products, your personal care products, your cookware, your furniture, your water. Most of them have never been tested in combination. We'll get into what the research actually says, which categories matter most, and the specific swaps that lower your toxic load without making you overhaul your whole life.

CHAPTER 4

The Chemical Environment

Here's something worth thinking about.

Your grandparents did not use nonstick cookware. They didn't have synthetic fragrances pumped through their HVAC systems. They didn't drink water that had traveled through plastic pipes, or store their food in plastic containers, or sleep in a bedroom with a Wi-Fi router on the nightstand and a phone charging two feet from their head.

None of those things existed.

Every single one of them is now standard in the modern home. And every single one of them is a chemical or electrical input your biology was never designed to process.

Here's where I want to be careful—because this topic goes wrong in two directions. Either people wave it off entirely—"everything causes cancer, nothing matters"—or they spiral into a fear-based obsession with scrubbing every possible toxin out of their life. Both of those miss the point.

Here's the point. Your body has a clearance capacity. It can handle a certain load of chemical exposure and process it out. The problem isn't that any single one of these exposures is going to destroy your health. The problem is that you're getting all of them—at once, continuously, from every direction—in a way that has never happened before in human history.

And when the load exceeds your clearance capacity, the system starts to fail. Not dramatically. Not all at once. Slowly, over years—and it shows up looking like a dozen different problems. Hormone disruption. Unexplained fatigue. Weight that won't move even though the diet is reasonable. Sleep that never fully restores. Inflammation that doesn't resolve.

This isn't detox culture. This is load mathematics.

And here's the part to really sit with. Your home, right now, is either lowering your biological load or raising it. There is no neutral. Every product you use, every material you cook in, every synthetic fragrance you breathe, every wireless signal running through your bedroom at night—these are all inputs. Your biology is processing them whether you're paying attention or not.

Now, the good news is you don't need a perfect environment. You need a lower-load one. You just need to bring the total input below your clearance threshold, and your body takes it from there. When the load drops, the nervous system downshifts. Fat becomes releasable—because fat-soluble toxins get stored in your fat tissue as a protective move, and your body holds on to that fat as long as the toxin burden stays high. Hormones stabilize. Sleep deepens.

There's a flip side to that, and it's worth knowing if you've ever tried to lose weight and stalled. Those fat-soluble compounds your body tucked away don't simply vanish—they come back out when the fat does. Lose fat slowly and your clearance systems can keep pace. Lose it fast, through crash diets or extreme calorie cutting, and you can release a wave of stored compounds back into your bloodstream faster than your liver and kidneys can process them. The chemicals measured climbing in the blood during rapid fat loss are exactly the fat-loving ones—PCBs, the old organochlorine pesticides, and their relatives.

This is one likely reason aggressive dieting so often backfires. It isn't only willpower, and it isn't only metabolism. So the order of operations matters: lower the incoming chemical load first, support the clearance pathways we just covered—the liver, plus water, fiber, and the cruciferous vegetables that help it work—and aim for steady fat loss instead of a sprint. You want the fat coming off at a rate your body can actually clean up after.

Not because you did some aggressive detox. Because you stopped pouring so much in.

Let me walk you through the four layers where this actually happens.

The first layer is the one that matters most—and the one people misunderstand the most. Endocrine disruptors.

These are compounds that interact with your hormonal system, not by adding hormones, but by mimicking them, blocking the receptor sites, or jamming the signal. They're signal mimics. And there are four big sources in the modern home.

Start with plastics. BPA is the one everybody's heard of, but phthalates—what's used to make plastic flexible, not that you needed the name—are arguably more concerning, and they're everywhere: food packaging, water bottles, the linings inside cans, the containers you heat food in. And here's the key: Heat speeds up the transfer of these compounds into your food and your liquid. So heating food in plastic—especially in a microwave—is not a minor exposure. It's a big one.

Then there's PFAS—the "forever chemicals." Nonstick cookware is the most direct source in most homes. They're called forever chemicals because they don't break down—not in the environment, and not well in your body either. They just accumulate. You'll also find them in waterproof clothing, food packaging, and some water supplies.

Synthetic fragrances surprise people. That one word—"fragrance"—on a product label is a legal umbrella that can hide hundreds of undisclosed compounds, most of them never tested for long-term biological effects. Air fresheners, scented candles, dryer sheets, most conventional cleaners, most conventional personal care products—that's continuous fragrance exposure. And boy, in a closed-up indoor space, that's a real daily chemical load most people never even think about.

And pesticides—both from your food and from indoor use. Glyphosate, which was originally patented as an antibiotic, now shows up in measurable amounts in the urine of most Americans. It was designed to kill microorganisms. And that is exactly what it does in your gut.

Put those four together, and here's what they do: They distort your thyroid signaling. They bias your body toward fat storage. They interfere with reproductive hormone production. They scramble the feedback loops your endocrine system uses to regulate itself. This is not a deficiency. It's signal interference. The machinery is all there—the signal coming into it is corrupted.

The second layer is the air and the water.

Indoor air is worse than outdoor air in most modern homes. And that's not an opinion—it's a consistent finding in the research. Sealed, insulated buildings trap volatile organic compounds off your furniture, your flooring, your paint, your cleaning products, your synthetic materials. Add synthetic fragrance, the combustion from cooking, and mold metabolites in any building with a moisture problem, and indoor air can run well above outdoor pollutant levels.

The fix here is simple and it costs nothing. Ventilation. Open the windows. Run the exhaust fans. Pull outdoor air through the space regularly. In a sealed modern building, that one habit makes a measurable difference.

Water is constant exposure—you contact it drinking, cooking, bathing, showering. The chlorine and chloramines used to treat municipal water are biologically active; they're antimicrobial agents, so they interact with your gut bacteria, and over the long term they can affect thyroid function. Fluoride, at high concentrations, is a thyroid disruptor. And microplastics now show up in virtually every municipal supply that's been tested.

So a good water filter on your drinking and cooking water is one of the highest-return investments you can make in this whole chapter. And shower filters matter too—your skin absorbs a lot during a hot shower, and breathing chlorine vapor in an enclosed shower is not a nothing exposure.

The third layer is heavy metals—and this is one most people don't think about at all. Lead, mercury, cadmium, arsenic. These aren't exotic industrial exposures. They're in old plumbing, certain fish, some cookware, certain foods.

What they do is inhibit your mitochondria, drive oxidative stress, and disrupt your enzymes. And here's the sneaky part: Heavy metals compete with your essential minerals at the receptor sites. Lead competes with calcium. Cadmium competes with zinc. So you can be eating plenty of zinc and still be functionally zinc-deficient, if your cadmium load is high enough to block it from getting in.

The strategy here is not aggressive chelation—that's an intervention with its own risks, and it belongs under medical supervision. The strategy is to reduce the exposure and support the exit routes. Which brings me to the most underrated idea in this entire chapter.

The fourth layer is the one almost nobody talks about. And it's the most important of all. Because the problem isn't only what comes in. It's what can't get out.

Your body has five exit routes for clearing chemical burden, and you want all five of them open.

The first is bile and the bowel. Your liver packages fat-soluble toxins into bile so they can be excreted. But if your bile flow is sluggish, or your bowel transit is slow, those toxins get reabsorbed instead of eliminated. This is why constipation isn't just a digestive inconvenience—it's a toxin-recirculation problem.

The second is your kidneys, and that one runs on hydration. Water-soluble compounds leave through your urine, and that takes adequate water. Get dehydrated, and clearance slows down.

The third is your skin, through sweat. Sweat is a badly underused exit route. Exercise that makes you sweat, and sauna use, both help clear compounds through the skin. That's real, it's measurable, and conventional medicine largely ignores it.

The fourth is your lungs. Some volatile compounds leave through your breath—and deep breathing and physical exertion help move them out.

And the fifth is your lymphatic system. Your lymph has no pump of its own—it depends entirely on muscle movement to keep flowing and carry waste toward elimination. Sit still all day and that route stagnates. Move, walk, and breathe deeply, and it keeps draining the way it's supposed to.

Here's what keeps all five of those routes open: magnesium, glycine—which you get from collagen—sulfur-containing foods like cruciferous vegetables and garlic and eggs, your B vitamins, and adequate trace minerals. These aren't detox supplements—they're the nutritional infrastructure that keeps the exit routes working. And when you're short on them—which most people are, as we covered back in Chapter 1—the routes slow down, and the load piles up faster.

Blocked exit routes plus continuous exposure equals a body stuck in chemical stress, with nowhere for that stress to go.

Now I want to talk about EMF—electromagnetic fields—directly, because this topic gets polarized fast. Either it's a massive threat, or it's complete pseudoscience. And the truth is more nuanced than either side.

Here's my honest take. The biological concern with EMF isn't mainly about high-intensity exposure cooking your tissue—that's the thermal argument, and the research there is genuinely mixed. The concern I find more credible is about chronic, low-level exposure, and what it does to your biological signaling over time.

Specifically, continuous EMF exposure may disrupt melatonin production, alter calcium signaling at the cellular level, fragment your sleep, and add to oxidative stress. These aren't dramatic, acute effects. They're cumulative and subtle—subtle enough that most people never connect their lousy sleep or their oxidative load to the wireless router they've been sleeping next to for five years.

And here's the key idea: with EMF, duration matters more than intensity. The quick exposure from running a microwave or walking past a cell tower isn't the issue. The issue is what's running continuously, at close range, for eight hours while you're trying to recover.

Which is why the bedroom is where this matters most. You spend roughly a third of your life in there. It's supposed to be your primary recovery environment. And running a Wi-Fi router, keeping a phone charging at arm's length, having devices humming on the nightstand all night—that's continuous low-level stimulation during the exact window your body needs to run its repair work.

Your body needs electrical quiet to signal safety—the same way it needs darkness, the same way it needs physical stillness. No organism recovers well under constant stimulation. That's not controversial. It's the same principle that explains why darkness improves sleep, and why chronic noise wrecks your health. The nervous system needs quiet in several dimensions at once.

I'm not telling you to throw your phone out the window. I'm telling you to get it out of your bedroom.

Now here's a connection most people have never heard—and it explains something that drives a lot of people crazy: they're doing everything right with their food, and the weight still won't move.

Fat-soluble toxins—persistent pollutants, certain pesticides, some heavy metals—get stored in your fat tissue. And that's actually a protective move. Your body is tucking these compounds away from your bloodstream, where they'd do more damage.

But here's the problem. Your body is reluctant to release fat that it's using as a storage vault for compounds it can't safely put back into circulation. If you drop fat fast while your toxic load is still high, you dump those stored compounds into your blood faster than you can clear them. And on some level, your body knows that. So fat loss slows down. Or it stops.

This is not a metabolism problem. It's a load problem.

And the fix is to work both ends at once. Lower the load coming in, while you support the exit routes going out. When your clearance capacity finally matches the burden, the fat becomes releasable again.

This is why some people find that once they clean up their chemical environment, weight loss that had been stuck for months suddenly starts moving again—with no change at all to their diet.

You don't need to overhaul your whole environment at once. You don't. You need three zones—and you start in this order.

Start with the bedroom. It's the highest return, because it's where you spend the most time, and where your recovery either happens or it doesn't. You want it dark, cool, fragrance-free, and low-EMF. Phone out of the room. Router off, or moved to another floor. And no synthetic fragrance anywhere in there—no air fresheners, no scented candles, no fragrance-heavy laundry products on your sheets. Redesign this one room, and you change the quality of the recovery that happens in it.

And it isn't only fragrance and signals in that room—it's the materials themselves. Conventional mattresses and memory foam can off-gas flame retardants and volatile organic compounds for years, and the same goes for synthetic carpet and brand-new furniture. You're breathing whatever the room is releasing for a third of your life, with your face right in it. When it's time to replace a mattress or bedding, look for certified low-emission or organic versions—and until then, air the room out whenever the weather lets you.

Then the kitchen. Stop heating food in plastic. Swap the nonstick cookware for stainless steel, cast iron, or ceramic. Run the exhaust fan when you cook—combustion byproducts build up fast in a closed kitchen. And filter your drinking and cooking water. These are changes you make once, and they keep paying off indefinitely.

Then the bathroom. Your conventional personal care products—shampoo, body wash, deodorant, lotion—are some of the highest daily chemical and fragrance exposures you've got. Switching to fragrance-free or genuinely clean versions cuts a major daily input most people never think about, only because it's been normal their entire life.

I want to be honest about something here, because I've made these mistakes myself.

Over the years I've done a lot of detox programs. And some of them put me in bed, genuinely sick, for two weeks. I didn't understand at the time that pulling too many toxins out too fast can trigger a serious immune reaction. Your body mobilizes stored compounds faster than it can clear them, and the result is not detox—it's a crisis.

I also went through a phase of getting paranoid about toxins. And I mean paranoid. Analyzing everything. Avoiding everything. You can take this so far that you end up living in a kind of bubble, and the stress of that—the vigilance, the constant checking—is probably doing as much damage as the toxins you're trying to avoid.

My thinking on this has shifted a lot over the years. On one hand, I do what I can to reduce exposure—the things we've covered in this chapter are real and worth doing. But on the other hand, it is impossible to be toxin-free. Welcome to planet Earth. Toxins exist. They always have. Your body was built for a certain amount of them.

What your body was not built for is a non-functional liver.

Your liver is your natural detoxifier—and the biochemistry

that breaks down chemical compounds into harmless particles needs as much attention as avoiding the chemicals in the first place. The best way to support it is straightforward: Make sure you have enough trace minerals—zinc, selenium, and the others—consume foods that support glutathione production (that's your master antioxidant), get sufficient quality protein from animal sources and fish, eat your cruciferous vegetables, and add fermented vegetables. My personal favorite is sauerkraut. I eat it regularly. It works.

Lower the load coming in. Keep the exit routes open. That's the whole strategy.

What to Actually Do

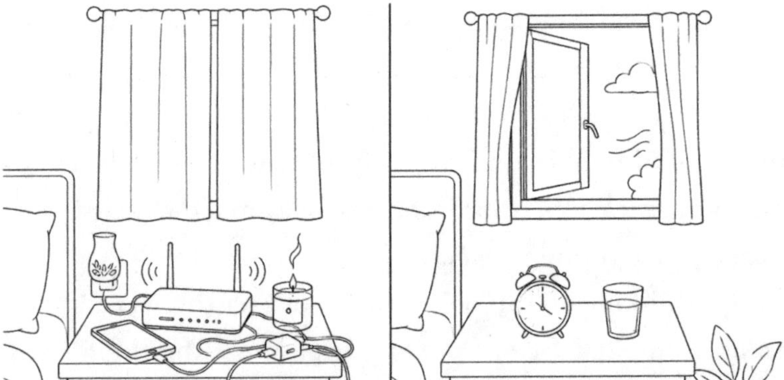

► START HERE

The one move that changes everything in Chapter 4:
Replace your nonstick cookware with stainless steel, cast-iron, or carbon steel. It costs under $50, it's permanent, and it removes your most direct daily PFAS exposure in one move. Do this before anything else in this chapter.

So here's how I'd sequence this—not all at once, in order of what actually moves the needle first.

1. **Get the phone out of the bedroom. Tonight.** It's free, it's immediate, and it fixes both the light problem from Chapter 2 and the EMF problem at the same time. Analog alarm clock. Phone charges in another room.
2. **Switch your cookware.** Nonstick out; cast-iron or stainless in. One-time purchase—and every meal you cook stops being a PFAS exposure.
3. **Filter your water.** Drinking and cooking water at the minimum. A decent countertop or under-sink carbon filter handles chlorine, chloramines, and most of the common contaminants.
4. **Get synthetic fragrance out of the bedroom and kitchen.** Scented candles, air fresheners, plug-ins—those are continuous chemical inputs in your highest-exposure rooms. Replace them with ventilation.
5. **Switch to fragrance-free personal care products.** Shampoo, body wash, deodorant. Read the labels—"fragrance" anywhere on the label means undisclosed

compounds. Pick products with full ingredient transparency.

6. **Open your windows daily.** Even fifteen minutes of ventilation per room makes a real difference in air quality. Costs nothing.
7. **Stock the exit-route foods so they're the default.** Eggs, garlic, and cruciferous vegetables give you the sulfur compounds that support phase 2 liver detox—the pathway that processes most fat-soluble compounds for elimination. Don't leave it to memory. Buy them every shop and keep them stocked in the fridge, so the supporting food is already in the house when you reach for something.
8. **Keep collagen or bone broth on hand.** Glycine—from collagen-rich foods like bone broth—is what your body uses to make glutathione, its main antioxidant and cleanup molecule, and most people on muscle-meat-heavy diets fall short. Keep broth in the freezer and a tub of collagen next to the kettle or the coffee, so it's the easy add rather than a project. Cheap, and it works.

The Fourteen-Day Chemical Reset

Week 1—Remove:

- All synthetic fragrance sources out of the house.
- Nonstick cookware replaced or set aside.
- Plastic food containers swapped for glass for hot food.
- Water filter installed or ordered.

- Bedroom: phone charging outside the room, any plug-in air fresheners removed.

Week 2—Reduce:

- Personal care products reduced to the lowest-ingredient versions you can find.
- Cleaning products replaced with single-ingredient alternatives.
- Bedroom aired out daily if weather allows.
- Any unnecessary chemical sources identified and removed.

Most people notice two things within fourteen days: better sleep quality—the bedroom burden drops first—and a subtle but real improvement in morning energy. Some notice that low-grade headaches, the kind they'd stopped attributing to anything, quietly disappear.

The Bottom Line

Your body is extraordinarily good at handling chemical exposure. It's got multiple layered systems—liver, kidneys, skin, lungs, gut—built specifically to process and clear out compounds that don't belong.

The problem is volume and continuity. The modern environment delivers chemical inputs from so many sources, continuously, that your clearance capacity gets overwhelmed. And it accumulates slowly, over years, and shows up as a dozen health problems that look unrelated.

The solution is not fear. It's not obsession. It's load reduction.

Lower what comes in. Support what goes out. Build three rooms that are genuinely low-threat. Your biology does the rest.

You don't need a perfect world. You need one safe zone to start. Then you expand from there.

The chemical environment's deepest effects land on the gut, where endocrine disruptors alter the microbiome you'll rebuild in Chapter 5—and the lowest-load room in the house should be the bedroom, which is exactly where this overlaps with the sleep environment from Chapter 2.

Next chapter: The Microbiome Environment. The 38 trillion microorganisms living in and on you are not passengers. They make neurotransmitters, they run a huge part of your immune system, they produce vitamins, they talk directly to your brain, and they decide whether the food you eat actually nourishes you or just passes through. The modern environment has done more damage to the microbiome in sixty years than the previous two hundred thousand—and most people have no idea it's even happening.

CHAPTER 5

The Microbiome Environment

► START HERE

The one move that unlocks everything in Chapter 5:

Add one serving of an unsweetened fermented food to your day—plain yogurt, kefir, sauerkraut, kimchi, or a spoonful of miso. Put it at the front of the fridge where you'll see it, the way you'd stock any staple. You're not taking a supplement; you're reseeding the ecosystem every single day with live microbes and the fiber they feed on. Do this before you change anything else in this chapter—a daily deposit of living cultures rebuilds gut diversity faster than anything you can remove. Start here.

Here's something that took me a long time to fully appreciate.

The 38 trillion microorganisms living in and on your body are not passengers. They're not hitchhikers you're putting up with. They're not some side issue in the story of your health.

They are, in many ways, running the show.

Your gut bacteria produce neurotransmitters—serotonin, dopamine, GABA. They train your immune system to tell the difference between a real threat and a harmless one. They make vitamins your body can't make on its own. They regulate inflammation. They talk directly to your brain through a dedicated nerve highway called the vagus nerve. And they decide whether the food you eat actually nourishes you or just passes through.

When that ecosystem is healthy, diverse, and balanced, most of the time you don't even know it's there. Everything just works.

When it collapses, nothing works quite right. And the modern environment has done more damage to the human microbiome in the last sixty years than in the previous two hundred thousand.

Honestly, I do not think we could live without our microbiome.

Now, I want to clear something up before we go any further, because the popular conversation about gut health gets this part wrong constantly.

The problem is not that you have bad bacteria. The problem is that you've lost diversity. You've lost the keystone species—"keystone" meaning the critical few that anchor the whole system. In the gut, it's those microbes that everything else depends on. And the "bad guys" that were always there in small numbers are allowed to overgrow when we lose these keystone microbes. The vast majority of good bacteria are the competition that keep them in check.

Think about a forest. A healthy forest has hundreds of species—trees, plants, fungi, insects, animals—all interacting, all keeping each other in check. Now come in and wipe out 60 percent of those species. What's left isn't just a smaller forest. It's an unstable one. The species that survive are the aggressive ones, the opportunists, the ones that grow fast in disturbed ground.

That's what antibiotic overuse, processed food, sterile living, and indoor life have done to your gut.

It's not a bad bacteria problem. It's an ecological gut environment collapse problem.

And you cannot fix an ecological collapse with a probiotic capsule. I want to be direct about that. Probiotics can help—I'm not dismissing them—but dropping a billion bacteria into a degraded environment that's missing its foundational diversity is not the same as rebuilding the ecosystem. You have to change the architecture.

So how did we lose this diversity? Let me walk you through it—because there isn't one cause. There are about five, and they've all been happening at the same time.

Start with antibiotics. They're the single biggest driver of microbiome disruption in modern life, and they get handed out like they're free.

Here's what a course of broad-spectrum antibiotics actually does to your gut. It's an ecological forest fire. It doesn't target the bad bacteria. It doesn't selectively pick off the ones causing trouble. It clears the forest. All of it. The keystone species, the beneficial organisms that took years to establish, the rare specialized bacteria that do jobs no supplement can replace—gone.

Your body does recover. But recovery is not automatic, and it's not complete. The studies on microbiome recovery after antibiotics show that some species never come back to their pre-antibiotic levels. The forest grows back—but boy, it's a different forest. Less diverse. More vulnerable to the next disruption.

One course as an adult is a significant event. Repeated

courses—which is the reality for most people who grew up in the last forty years—can leave you with a chronically simplified ecosystem that never fully stabilizes.

And then there's the antibiotics given in childhood, when the microbiome was still being built. The first three years of life are the critical window for immune programming—the gut is learning what's foreign and what's not, what to attack and what to tolerate. Disrupt that window with antibiotics, and the immune miscalibration that results can last for decades. Allergies, autoimmune conditions, food sensitivities—those aren't random. They're often the signature of early ecological disruption.

Then there's the food itself. And here's something that doesn't get talked about enough: Food used to be alive.

Not in a mystical sense. Literally. Ancestral food—vegetables pulled out of the soil, fermented foods, raw dairy, naturally aged products—carried environmental microorganisms. Soil bacteria. Lactobacillus from fermentation. Diverse organisms that had been living on the surface of the plants. So when you ate that food, you were continuously replenishing your microbial ecosystem from the environment.

Even the great majority of vegetables and salad you buy in the grocery store is grown hydroponically—without soil. The soil is what gives the plant its microbes. Maybe you never considered your vegetables as probiotics, but they are filled inside and out with microbes—this is not a bad thing.

Modern food is sterilized. Pasteurized, irradiated, preserved, packaged—every microbial organism eliminated. It's shelf-stable and sterile and nutritionally depleted and ecologically empty. When you eat it, you're taking in fuel. You're not taking in any microbial input.

So the ecosystem gets no replenishment. It slowly simplifies. The species that needed regular reinforcement from environmental exposure start to decline.

Fermented foods—sauerkraut, kefir, kimchi, aged cheese, yogurt with live cultures—were in virtually every traditional diet on earth. Not because our ancestors understood lactobacillus. Because the food naturally fermented, and they ate it.

Now here's one that sounds completely backward: Being too clean is making us sick.

I'm not saying dirty is healthy. I'm not saying hygiene doesn't matter. I'm being specific. Your immune system needs microbial exposure to calibrate correctly. It's a training system, and it needs something to train against. When kids grow up with minimal soil contact, no animal exposure, antibacterial everything, and highly sanitized indoor environments—the immune system doesn't get the training it needs.

And what happens to an immune system with nothing real to respond to? It starts responding to things it shouldn't. Pollen. Food proteins. Its own tissues. Allergies, food sensitivities, autoimmune conditions—the rates of all of these have risen sharply in exactly the countries and time periods where sanitation and indoor living became standard. That is not a coincidence.

There's a reason farm kids have lower rates of asthma and allergies than city kids. There's a reason kids with pets have more robust immune profiles than kids without. There's a reason the kids who play in the dirt are, in the ways that matter, healthier for it.

The immune system needs early microbial input. And we've cut it off.

Then there's what ultra-processed food does from the inside. The emulsifiers, the preservatives, the stabilizers—they do something most people have no idea about.

Compounds like polysorbate 80 and carboxymethylcellulose—common additives, not that you needed the names—don't just mess with your metabolism. They degrade the mucosal layer that lines your gut. That layer is the barrier between your gut contents and your bloodstream. And it's also the habitat for a specific set of bacteria that live right at the gut wall and are critical for keeping that barrier intact.

When emulsifiers break down that mucosal layer, the bacteria living there lose their home. The barrier gets more permeable—what most people call "leaky gut." And your immune system, which is supposed to be walled off from your gut contents by that barrier, starts running into things it was never meant to see. That's a recipe for chronic, low-grade inflammation.

And this is separate from what these foods do to your insulin. They're doing both at once. The metabolic disruption and the microbial disruption are happening at the same time, feeding each other.

And then there's the other side of the food problem—what you're not feeding them.

Here's the thing. Your gut bacteria don't eat what you eat.

They eat what you don't digest. Specifically: diverse plant fibers, and polyphenols that make it past your small intestine and reach the colon, where the bulk of your microbiome actually lives.

Feed them a wide range of plant fibers, and you get a diverse microbiome. Feed them processed grain fiber—the main "healthy fiber" in most modern diets—and you get a simplified monoculture. The species that thrive on grain fiber outcompete everything else, and the specialists that need the fibers from tubers, wild plants, legumes, and varied vegetables die off.

The diversity of what you eat directly determines the diversity of who lives in your gut.

And the standard modern diet—even a "healthy" one—is monotonous compared to what a human gut ecosystem actually needs. Twenty to thirty different plant foods a week would be a great target. Most people eat three to five. And fermented foods add both prebiotics (food for microbes) and probiotics.

I want to spend a minute on why this matters way beyond digestion—because most people file the microbiome under "gut issue." It is not a gut issue.

Start with your immune system. Roughly 70 to 80 percent of your immune tissue sits in or right next to your gut. And the microbiome directly trains those immune responses—teaching the system what to attack and what to leave alone. When the ecosystem is disrupted, immune miscalibration follows. The system becomes either hyperreactive—allergies, autoimmunity, food sensitivities—or underreactive—recurrent infections, poor surveillance. And both can show up in the same person.

Then there's mental health. Your gut produces about 90 percent of your body's serotonin. Not in the brain—in the gut, largely by your gut bacteria. And that vagus nerve, the direct line between gut and brain, carries more signals up to the brain than down from it. So when the ecosystem is disrupted, neurotransmitter production gets disrupted. The connection between gut dysbiosis and depression, anxiety, and brain fog is now one of the most actively researched areas in all of medicine. This isn't fringe. It's mainstream.

Then there's nutrient production. Your gut bacteria make vitamin K2, several of the B vitamins, and short-chain fatty acids—especially butyrate, which is the main fuel for the cells lining your colon. So without a healthy microbiome, you can be eating a nutritionally complete diet and still be functionally deficient—because the production side is broken.

And then there's inflammation. A disrupted microbiome is a pro-inflammatory microbiome. That chronic, low-grade inflammation—the kind that sits underneath cardiovascular disease, metabolic syndrome, cognitive decline, most of the chronic conditions—is strongly tied to microbiome disruption. And it runs both ways: Inflammation also disrupts the microbiome. But the gut is very often where the cycle starts.

Here's a practical point that connects to everything above, and most people never hear it. Your stomach acid is part of this system.

Stomach acid is your first line of ecological defense. It kills pathogens before they ever reach the intestine. It creates the acidic environment that controls what survives the trip from your mouth to your gut. It's the gatekeeper.

When your stomach acid is low—from stress, from antacid use, from proton pump inhibitor medications—organisms that should have been killed in the stomach survive and make it into the small intestine. And the small intestine is not designed to house large bacterial populations. When they accumulate there, you get what's commonly called SIBO—small intestinal bacterial overgrowth. Bloating, gas, food intolerances, poor nutrient absorption.

PPIs—the proton pump inhibitors, the acid-blocking drugs—are among the most prescribed medications in the world. And they have their place. But long-term use in people who don't have a serious medical reason for them is an ecological intervention, with downstream consequences most prescribing doctors never discuss.

Low stomach acid also means poor protein digestion. And undigested protein reaching the colon gets fermented by the wrong organisms, producing compounds that irritate the gut lining even more.

The gut ecology depends on the stomach doing its job.

Now, I want to be honest here about my own experience with this, because I got it wrong for a long time.

I had gut issues for years that I couldn't fully resolve. I tried elimination diets. I tried various protocols. Some of them helped, partially. None of them fixed it completely.

What actually shifted things for me was simpler than any protocol. I started eating sauerkraut every day. Not a supplement. Not ten cups of spinach. Not a capsule. Real, naturally fermented sauerkraut—the kind with live cultures, not the pasteurized stuff sitting on the regular grocery shelf.

Within a few weeks, the bloating I'd had for years started clearing up. My digestion improved noticeably. And I started to notice the difference between the days I ate it and the days I didn't.

Now I eat it every day. It's not exciting. It doesn't require a protocol or a schedule. You just eat it.

And here's what I think happened. I'd been feeding the ecosystem supplements while starving it of what it actually needed—continuous ecological replenishment from live fermented food, the way human guts were replenished for two hundred thousand years before we sterilized everything.

What to Actually Do

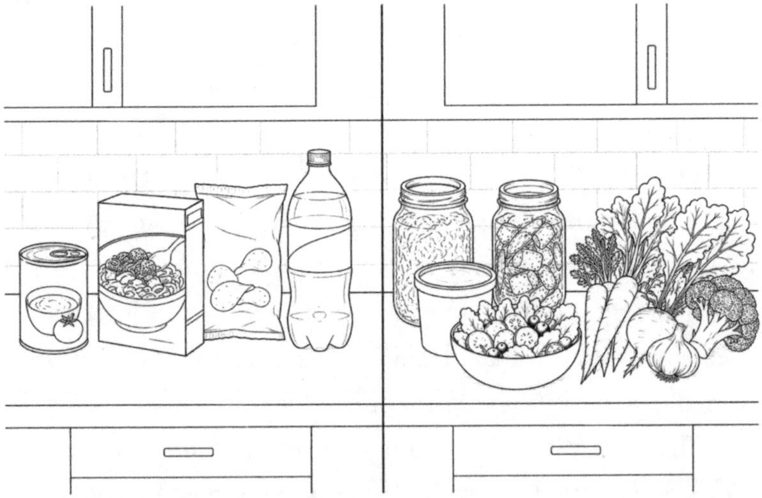

So here's how you actually restore the ecosystem—and notice, none of this is a protocol. It's just giving the ecosystem back what it's been missing.

1. **Keep live fermented food in the fridge so it's already there.** Sauerkraut is the easiest way in—real sauerkraut, refrigerated, with live cultures, not the shelf-stable pasteurized jar. Don't make it a daily decision: keep an open jar in the fridge so a forkful with a meal takes no thought. This is continuous ecological replenishment, not a supplement protocol. Kefir, kimchi, plain yogurt with live cultures, and aged cheeses all count too—keep a couple on hand and rotate between them.
2. **Diversify the cart, not your willpower at the table.** The lever here is what goes in the cart, because what's in the house is what gets eaten. Count how many different plant foods you eat in a week; the target is twenty to thirty, and if it's under twenty, widen the rotation—buy a different vegetable or two every shop, mix colors and textures, swap things in rather than repeating the same five. This doesn't mean eating foods you hate. Each different plant fiber feeds a different set of gut bacteria. Diversity in, diversity out. One caveat: If you have active, significant gut inflammation, a lot of fiber can aggravate it in the short term. Some people do better temporarily easing off fiber—even down to a low-fiber or carnivore-style approach—to let the gut lining settle, then reintroducing plant diversity as it heals. If that's you, work it out with a clinician rather than self-diagnosing, and treat it as a temporary step, not the destination.
3. **Reduce antibiotics to necessary use only.** This is not a recommendation to skip them when you actually need

them—that's a different and serious problem. But taking antibiotics for a viral infection, which they don't treat, or for something that would clear on its own, is an ecological event with lasting consequences. Have that conversation with your doctor.

4. **If you've had significant antibiotic exposure, support the recovery on purpose.** Fermented foods, plus diverse plant fiber, plus time. Don't expect your microbiome to rebuild itself on a standard Western diet. The ecosystem needs substrate and replenishment at the same time.
5. **Get outside and get your hands dirty once in a while.** Gardening. Hiking. Soil contact. Animal contact. Environmental microbial exposure isn't a risk—it's ecological input your immune system needs. The obsession with sanitizing every surface and avoiding all microbial contact is immunologically counterproductive.
6. **Protect your stomach acid.** If you're on acid-blocking medication long-term and you don't have a documented reason that requires it, that's worth a conversation with your doctor. Stomach acid is ecological infrastructure—reducing it has downstream consequences.
7. **Keep broth and organ meats stocked.** Like we covered in Chapter 1—but here's the gut connection: The glycine from collagen supports the mucosal gut lining directly. That lining turns over fast and needs continuous nutritional support, and glycine is one of the key substrates. Keep bone broth in the freezer and liver in there too, so the resilience-building food is already on hand. It's

why traditional diets that included collagen-rich foods produced more gut resilience than the modern muscle-meat-only diet.

The Bottom Line

Your microbiome is not a supplement category. It's an ecosystem.

And ecosystems don't respond to supplementation when the architecture is wrong. They respond to restoration—to getting back the conditions that let the ecosystem flourish in the first place. Diverse food. Ecological exposure. Live fermented food. Protection from unnecessary antibiotics. And a gut terrain that can actually support microbial life.

Modern life removed most of those conditions all at once. And the result is a simplified, fragile gut ecosystem that's reactive, inflammatory, and not doing the jobs it was designed to do.

You don't need a complex protocol. You need to restore the basics: diverse plant food, fermented food daily, less sterile living, and protection of the terrain.

The ecosystem knows what to do. Give it what it needs, stop taking away what it requires, and it will start to restore itself.

Your microbiome is a hub, not a side room. It turns the food from Chapter 1 into the building blocks and neurotransmitters that shape your nutrient status (Chapter 9) and your mood and focus (Chapter 6). Feed the microbes well and several environments improve at once.

Next chapter: The Cognitive Environment. Your attention isn't really yours anymore—it's being actively competed for by systems built specifically to capture it and hold it. The dopamine hijack running through every screen, every notification, every algorithmically optimized feed is doing something measurable to your brain's reward circuitry. We'll get into what the research actually shows, why boredom is not a problem you need to solve, and how to redesign your cognitive environment so your mind is working for you instead of being worked on.

CHAPTER 6

The Cognitive Environment

> ► **START HERE**
>
> **The one move that unlocks everything in Chapter 6:**
> Turn off every notification that isn't a real human being contacting you directly. Open your settings now and kill the badges, banners, and buzzes for everything else—news, social, games, shopping, "someone you may know." Your attention isn't leaking because you're weak; it's being pulled by design. Cut the signals at the source and the phone stops reaching into your focus dozens of times a day. This one change defends your attention with no willpower required. Start here.

I spend more than eight hours a day on a computer.

Heavy cognitive focus. Researching health data, reading biochemistry journals, cross-referencing studies, writing. Day after day. I genuinely love it—this is not a complaint. But here's what I've noticed: When I finally stop and go outside for a walk, I'm still not outside.

My body is walking. I am still in my head. Still running the problem I was working on. Still processing the last study I read. I'm physically present in a field in the sun, and mentally I'm still at my desk.

It takes me over an hour of walking to actually extract my attention from inside my skull and land it in my environment.

One hour. Just to stop thinking.

Now if that's happening to me—and I know exactly what's going on neurologically, and I'm actively trying to stop—imagine what's happening to someone who doesn't know, isn't trying, and has seven different notification systems running simultaneously on their phones.

That's what this chapter is about.

Here's the mainstream position on focus and attention problems: You need more discipline. Better habits. A stricter schedule. Maybe medication if it's bad enough.

That is so not true.

The problem is not discipline. The problem is that your cognitive environment is running a load your brain was never designed to handle—and it's doing it continuously, with no off switch, and no recovery window built in.

Your brain evolved to handle one problem at a time. Real, physical problems. Find food. Navigate terrain. Solve an immediate social conflict. Then rest. Then the next problem.

What it did not evolve for: forty-seven browser tabs. Three hundred unread emails. Slack pinging every four minutes. A news feed algorithmically optimized to keep your amygdala activated. A phone that buzzes eighty times a day. And after all of that—a streaming service with ten thousand options waiting to fill whatever cognitive space might have been left over.

The average person now receives sixty-five to eighty smartphone notifications per day. They switch tasks every forty-seven seconds on average during computer work. After an interruption, it takes an average of twenty-three minutes to return to full focus on the original task.

Do that math. If you're interrupted every forty-seven seconds, you never return to full focus. Not once during the entire workday.

That's not a discipline problem. That's an attention scattering problem.

Here's something most people get wrong, and it explains a lot. I want to get into a little biology for a minute.

Dopamine is not the pleasure chemical. That's serotonin. Dopamine is the pursuit chemical. It's the signal that fires when your brain identifies something worth going after. It creates motivation, drive, forward movement toward apparent survival. It's what gets you out of bed, keeps you working on something hard, makes you feel like the effort is worth it.

When dopamine fires correctly—in response to real effort, real progress, real reward—it's one of the most important systems in your body. It's why humans accomplish anything at all.

Now here's what the modern environment did to it.

Every notification is a small dopamine hit. Every scroll produces a hit. Every like, every update, every algorithmically selected piece of content that matches your specific emotional triggers—hit, hit, hit. Small ones. Cheap ones. Effortless ones.

And here's the problem: when dopamine fires too often, too easily, with too little effort—the brain protects itself by reducing receptor sensitivity. It downregulates. The same signal produces less response. So it takes more input to get the same feeling.

This is the exact same mechanism behind tolerance in addiction. When the initial pleasure gets lost and you need more and more of it to get pleasure.

The result: Real life starts to feel flat. Reading a book—which produces slow, effortful, low-frequency dopamine—feels boring compared to a feed that produces rapid-fire hits. A real conversation feels dull. Deep work feels impossible to start. The motivation system has been recalibrated to respond to cheap, fast inputs—and everything else gets filtered out as not worth the effort.

And here's what makes this worse: After roughly thirty days of chronic overstimulation, measurable changes in dopamine receptor density show up in brain imaging. This is not a mood. It's a structural shift. It takes sixty to ninety days of reduced stimulation to meaningfully reverse it.

That's two to three months to recalibrate what the environment is doing to you daily.

These systems were designed by some of the best engineers on Earth with one specific goal: maximum time and attention on a platform. Not your well-being. Not your productivity. Not your relationships. Time on a platform. That metric drives revenue.

Infinite scroll was invented specifically to remove natural stopping points. Before infinite scroll, you'd reach the bottom of a page and make a decision: keep going or stop. Infinite scroll eliminated the stopping cue. There is no bottom.

Our environment has been engineered for hijacking attention.

Autoplay was designed to remove endings. You finish one video—the natural completion point where a person would stop—and the next one starts in three seconds. The decision to continue is replaced with friction to stop.

Variable reward is the slot machine mechanism. You don't get a hit every time you scroll. Sometimes it's nothing, sometimes it's something interesting, occasionally it's something that really gets you. Unpredictable reward is more addictive than predictable reward—that's established behavioral science, and these platforms use it deliberately.

The algorithm knows you. Not generally—specifically. It has enough behavioral data on you to know what makes you angry, what makes you anxious, what makes you click, what keeps you scrolling at 11:00 p.m. when you should be sleeping. And it optimizes for those triggers automatically, millions of times per second, individually tailored.

Your willpower evolved to handle finite temptation with clear endings. It did not evolve for infinite, personalized, engineered extraction with no stopping point.

You cannot out-discipline this. Your environment has to change.

Of course there is one exception: Dr. Berg YouTube videos—addiction to those is totally okay.

Not all bad habits are equal. Here is the honest truth about what damages your dopamine system the most: **Internet pornography is number one.**

Most health books avoid saying this directly, but it is uniquely destructive because it combines four things:

- **Extreme novelty** (always something new to see)
- **Sexual wiring** (hijacks your brain's strongest natural drives)
- **Zero effort** (instantly available)
- **Infinite escalation** (you can keep looking for more extreme content)

Because of this combo, it burns out your brain's dopamine receptors faster and harder than almost any other behavior. In fact, regular use can physically alter your brain structure in just a few months.

Once you quit, it takes at least **sixty to ninety days** for your brain to reset. If you don't fix this habit first, none of the other health advice will work. It has to be your top priority.

Short-form video feeds are second. TikTok, Instagram Reels, YouTube Shorts. These are variable reward machines optimized for the shortest possible dopamine cycle—three to fifteen seconds per hit, infinite continuation, zero effort, no completion. The average TikTok user opens the app eight times per day and spends ninety minutes on it. When I see someone scrolling through shorts, I always ask them, *Did you get to the end yet?*

High-frequency notifications are third. The average smartphone user checks their phone ninety-six times per day—once every ten minutes during waking hours. Each check is a dopamine trigger whether there's anything there or not. The anticipation is the dopamine hit. Most people have given forty to sixty apps automatic permission to interrupt them at any moment.

Binge streaming, outrage news cycles, and reward-loop gaming are the next tier. Each one has the same architecture: no natural ending, variable reward, emotional activation. Stacked together—which is how most people use them—the combined load is significant.

The key word is *stacked*. It's not one of these. It's all of them running simultaneously, every day, with no recovery window built in.

Here's where most people miss the connection. They think this is a productivity problem, or a focus problem. It's a whole-body problem.

When your brain interprets an unresolved notification loop, an open task pile, and constant context switching as unresolved threat—and it does, because that's how the nervous system categorizes unresolved demands—cortisol rises.

Not the acute cortisol of a real emergency that gets metabolized through physical movement the way we discussed in Chapter 3. Chronic, low-grade cortisol. The kind that stays elevated from morning to night without ever discharging.

That chronic cortisol degrades sleep quality—which means the light clock from Chapter 2 never fully resets. Poor sleep elevates ghrelin, your hunger hormone, making the food environment from Chapter 1 harder to navigate. Elevated cortisol increases inflammatory load that adds to the chemical burden from Chapter 4. And a chronically stressed nervous system degrades gut motility and stomach acid production—which disrupts the microbiome from Chapter 5.

Cognitive overload is not isolated in the brain. It cascades everywhere.

There's also something happening at the brain level specifically: Chronic high cortisol measurably shrinks the hippocampus—the memory and learning center—over time. It impairs prefrontal cortex function, which is where decision-making, impulse control, and long-term thinking happen. The irony: the cognitive overload that's supposed to make you more productive makes you less productive.

I want to be honest about my own experience here, because it's directly relevant.

Personally, I spend easily eight-plus hours a day of intense cognitive work. Researching, reading, writing about health—day after day. I like it. I'm not complaining about the work itself.

But what I noticed was that when I finally went outside—which I do every single day, minimum two hours, no phone—I wasn't actually outside. I was still inside my head. Still running the last problem. Still processing. My body had changed locations, but my brain hadn't.

And here's what I learned: It takes me over an hour of walking before my attention actually extracts from my own head and lands in my environment. One hour before I can actually see what's around me. Before I notice the trees. Before the problems stop running.

When I first started doing this deliberately—going outside with no phone, no podcast, no music even—it felt like wasted time.

But it is the opposite of wasted time. It turned out to be the most productive thing I do every day now.

Because here's what I eventually realized: The two hours outside wasn't recovery from the work. It was required for the work. The creativity, insights that would take me hours of grinding to reach at my desk—they'd arrive on the walk. Effortlessly. Because I'd finally given my mind the unstructured time it needed to process what it had absorbed.

Don't make the mistake I made for years—thinking that more hours at the desk means more production. It doesn't. The off time is doing work you can't do consciously.

This is the most counterintuitive thing in this chapter, so I'm going to say it plainly.

Boredom is not a problem to solve. Boredom is the recovery state. Think about why people stay on social media—to never get bored—constant entertainment.

The modern reflex is to eliminate boredom the instant it appears. Waiting room—pull out the phone. Walking the dog—earbuds in. Cooking dinner—TV on in the background. Driving—podcast. Every gap, every moment of potential quiet, filled immediately.

There are no gaps. There is no quiet. And as a result, there is no recovery.

Here's what your brain actually does during unstructured, unstimulated time: it consolidates (combines and makes stronger) memories from the day. It connects information across different things that were processed in separate sessions. It resets baseline dopamine sensitivity which directly affects creativity, self-reflection, future planning, and insight generation.

When you never give it quiet, it never gets to do its work.

I am genuinely recommending that you make time to be bored every day. Schedule twenty minutes of nothing. Sit outside with no phone. Walk without audio. Do a physical task with no background media. Stare at something that isn't a screen.

It's harder than it seems. At first it could take two hours to activate this "turn off" switch.

The discomfort you feel at first—that pull to fill the silence, that low-level anxiety about not being productive—that's your dopamine system trying to recalibrate and being interrupted by your own reflex to avoid discomfort.

Be comfortable with the discomfort. It resolves within one to two weeks for most people. What's on the other side of it is something that used to be normal and now feels remarkable: a mind that can actually rest.

This will save you from burnout. I've seen it in my own life and in the people I work with. The ones who burn out are not the ones who work the hardest. They're the ones who never stop.

Here's a framing shift that pulls everything together.

You redesigned your food environment so the right choice is the easy choice. You fixed the light environment so the timing system gets the right signal. You reduced the chemical load in your home. Same logic applies here.

Your cognitive environment—your phone, your apps, your

notification settings, your default media consumption—is an environment. It either supports your brain or degrades it. There is no neutral.

And just like the food environment, the solution is not willpower. It's architecture. You design it once, correctly, and it runs in your favor automatically.

What does a well-designed cognitive environment look like?

No infinite scroll apps on your phone. Not hidden in a folder—deleted. A folder still has zero friction. Deletion means the decision was made once, permanently, in a moment of clear thinking rather than renegotiated at 10:00 p.m. when your resistance is lowest.

Notifications off by default for everything except calls. Every app that wants to interrupt you has to earn that access. Most of them haven't. Revoke it from all of them and add it back only to the ones that genuinely require real-time attention.

Phone charges in another room. Every night. The bedroom is a recovery environment. A phone on the nightstand is a cognitive intrusion device sitting two feet from your head during the only time your brain gets to fully rest.

One deep work block daily with the phone physically in another room. Not face down on the desk. In another room. Research on this is consistent: The mere presence of a smartphone on a desk—even face down, even off—measurably reduces available cognitive capacity. The brain allocates resources to not checking it. Remove the temptation entirely, and those resources go to the work.

What to Actually Do

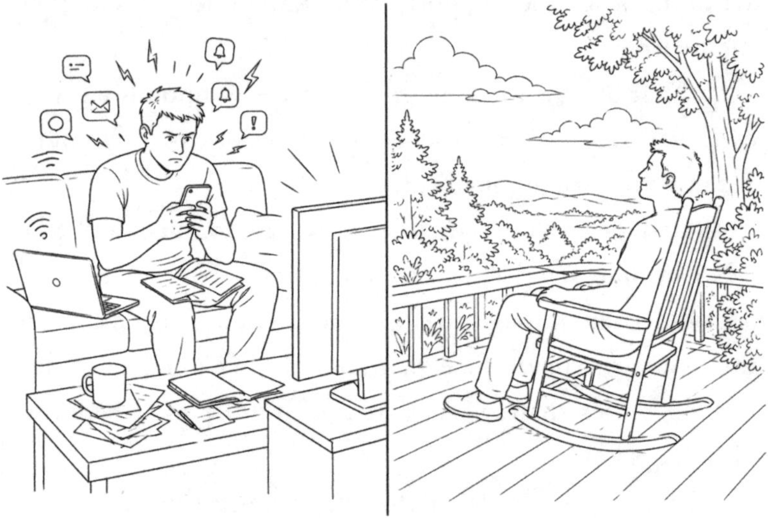

So here's how I'd sequence it—in order of impact.

1. **Get the phone out of the bedroom. Tonight.** Analog alarm clock. Phone charges in another room. This is nearly free, immediate, and addresses the light problem from Chapter 2 and the cognitive problem simultaneously.
2. **Protect the first thirty to sixty minutes of your morning.** No phone, no news, no social media—real-world sensory input before digital input. You already set this up by charging the phone in another room; the move now is simply not going to get it. Don't carry it to the coffee or the kitchen table. This one habit changes the quality of your attention for the entire day. The first

thing your brain processes in the morning sets the baseline for everything that follows.

3. **Turn off all notifications.** All of them. Go into settings right now and turn off every notification from every app. Then add back only what genuinely requires real-time access. You'll add back maybe three things. Everything else was interrupting you by default because you never opted out.
4. **Delete infinite scroll apps.** Not moderation. Deletion. If the app has no natural ending, it doesn't belong on your phone. The decision gets made once, clearly, and then the architecture enforces it without requiring daily willpower.
5. **Disable autoplay everywhere.** YouTube, Netflix, every streaming platform. Endings must exist. The completion signal—that's done, I'm choosing to stop—is a cognitive stopping cue that autoplay removes on purpose. Put it back.
6. **Schedule twenty minutes of nothing, daily.** Pick a spot where screens don't go—a chair on the deck, the porch, a bench—and give it a fixed slot. Twenty minutes there with no phone, no audio, no input: sit, rock, walk, watch something that isn't a screen. You're not summoning discipline; you've built a place with nothing to scroll, so boredom—the recovery state—happens on its own. The discomfort at first is the recalibration beginning. Stay with it.
7. **Leave the device behind so the silent walk is the only walk.** No podcast, no music, no calls—soft

environmental attention, noticing what's around you, letting your mind wander without directing it. Don't decide this at the door every time. Set it up so it's automatic: earbuds in a bowl by the door, phone left on the charger. If the audio isn't on you, the quiet walk is the only one available. At least four times a week. This produces a cognitive reset that is qualitatively different from any other intervention in this list. Your nervous system needs actual sensory contact with the real world. Not a screen version of nature. The real thing.

8. **Put friction on the reward so effort comes first.** Work first, then entertainment. Movement first, then the podcast. Deep-work block first, then the video. Don't police the order in the moment—build it in. Stay logged out of the entertainment apps, keep the game controller in a drawer, so the reward takes a few steps to reach and the effort is the easier thing to start. This restores the effort-to-reward sequence dopamine evolved for. Reward without effort desensitizes the system. Reward after effort strengthens it.

The Bottom Line

The modern cognitive environment is running a biological mismatch.

Your brain evolved for one problem at a time, natural endings, silence between tasks, and effort-based reward. It did not evolve for eighty notifications a day, infinite scroll, algorithmically optimized emotional activation, and zero unstructured time.

The result is a dopamine system recalibrated to cheap, fast inputs, a nervous system that can't find an off switch, and a mind that can't stop even when the body has left the building—which is exactly what I experience every time it takes me an hour of walking to stop thinking.

That's not a personal failing. That's the architecture working exactly as designed—for the platform, not for you.

Change the architecture. Protect the quiet. Schedule the boredom. Let the recalibration happen.

And go outside without your phone. Every single day if you can manage it. The two hours I spend outside daily aren't time away from my work. They're what makes the work possible.

Your brain knows how to rest. It just needs you to stop filling every moment it tries to.

The dopamine environment loops straight back through the others. The same screens that fracture your focus also delay your sleep (Chapter 2) and pull you toward late-night eating (Chapter 1)—and they quietly crowd out the real social connection coming up in Chapter 7.

Next chapter: The Social Architecture. The people around you are an environment—and the research on what chronic loneliness, toxic relationships, and social disconnection do to your biology is as concrete as anything we've covered. We'll look at what unsafe social environments do to cortisol, immune function, and lifespan—and how to design the social environment the same way you've been designing all the others.

CHAPTER 7

The Social Environment

> ► **START HERE**
>
> **The one move that unlocks everything in Chapter 7:**
>
> Put one unhurried, in-person connection on your calendar every week—and make it recurring, not "sometime soon." A standing walk with a friend, a weekly meal, a phone-free coffee with someone who restores you rather than drains you. Connection fades not because you stopped caring but because nothing in your week protects it. Give it a fixed slot the way you'd protect any appointment, and the relationship stops depending on who happens to reach out. Start here.

Here's something that will probably surprise you.

Loneliness is not an emotion.

It's a threat signal.

Your brain processes social isolation the same way it processes physical danger. Not metaphorically—the same neural circuitry, the same stress chemistry, the same cascade of cortisol and inflammatory compounds that fire when you're in genuine physical danger. Your nervous system cannot tell the difference between being alone and being at risk. For most of human history, those two things were the same.

A person separated from the tribe didn't survive long. So the brain evolved to treat isolation as an emergency. And it still does—even when you're sitting alone in a perfectly comfortable apartment, with food in the fridge and the door locked.

That response doesn't care about your circumstances. It cares about one question it's asking constantly, underneath everything else you're thinking and feeling:

Am I protected by others?

If yes—cortisol drops. Inflammation quiets. Digestion improves. Sleep deepens. Repair activates. The body gets the signal that it's okay to stop defending and start recovering.

If no—defense mode stays on. Stress chemistry persists. Healing suppresses. The body keeps its resources allocated to survival rather than repair.

This is not psychology. This is autonomic biology. And the modern social environment is getting the answer wrong for more people than at any point in human history.

The standard advice on loneliness and social connection goes like this: make more friends, join groups, put yourself out there, be more open. It treats connection as a personality challenge. Something you work on. A skill to develop.

That is so not true.

Connection is not a personality challenge. It's a biological requirement—like food, like light, like movement. You don't tell someone with a vitamin D deficiency to just "try harder to absorb sunlight." You fix the environment that's blocking them from getting what they need.

The same logic applies here. If your social environment isn't delivering what your nervous system requires, the solution is not to become a more social person. It's to redesign the environment.

And right now, for most people, the architecture is broken in ways they can't even see—because the replacement looks so much like the real thing.

Let me explain the biology first, because once you understand it, everything else in this chapter makes immediate sense.

Oxytocin is commonly called the love hormone. That's not quite right. Oxytocin is the anti-cortisol (anti-stress) hormone.

Here's what it actually does: it blocks cortisol receptors. Directly. When oxytocin is present, cortisol cannot fully bind. Blood pressure drops. Inflammation decreases. Heart rate slows. Pain tolerance increases. The nervous system receives a direct chemical signal that says: You are not alone, stand down.

Without sufficient oxytocin input—not occasionally, but regularly, repeatedly, in sufficient doses—the stress system dominates by default. Not because something bad happened. Because the off switch for the stress response requires oxytocin to activate, and the oxytocin isn't coming.

You can eat perfectly. Sleep eight hours. Exercise daily. Take every supplement on your list. And still have chronic elevated cortisol, persistent inflammation, and a nervous system that never fully settles—because the social environment isn't delivering what the chemistry requires.

This is not a mood problem. It's a deficiency state. The same way iron deficiency produces anemia regardless of how much sleep you get, oxytocin deficiency produces a chronic stress state regardless of how clean your diet is.

Now here's what actually triggers oxytocin release—and this is where the modern social environment fails most dramatically.

Physical touch of at least twenty seconds. Eye contact. Hearing a real human voice—not scrolling social media. Shared physical activity. Shared meals without distraction. Animal (pet) interaction. These are the primary inputs.

What does not trigger meaningful oxytocin release: texting, social media, scrolling through other people's faces, Zoom calls in most contexts, likes, comments, followers, messages.

Digital contact stimulates. It does not regulate.

Your nervous system evolved to receive connection signals through PHYSICAL presence—eye contact, voice tone, micro-expressions, touch, proximity. It cannot extract the same signal via a screen or experiencing sex through a porno video. It's like trying to get vitamin D from a photograph of the sun.

I want to tell you about a close relative. I'll keep it vague enough to protect her privacy, but the details matter, so I'm going to be specific.

She had terrible acne. Not occasional breakouts—persistent, severe acne that had devastated her self-esteem over months. We worked on it hard. A diet overhaul, detox, and different foods to avoid allergies. A nutrient protocol—B-complex, zinc, everything that should have moved the needle. All the usual recommendations. All of it.

Nothing worked. I was baffled.

Then one day she told me her skin had completely cleared up. She sent me pictures. And boy, I could not believe the difference. Complete transformation.

Of course I asked: What the heck did you do right before it cleared up?

She said: I found several new wonderful friends. We've been hanging out every night, laughing until the early hours of the morning.

What?

Staying up into the night?

Yes.

Wild!

She had been lonely for months. And it showed up in her skin.

Now think about what was actually happening biologically. Months of chronic loneliness—cortisol elevated, inflammation running continuously, the stress system never fully discharging. Acne is an inflammatory condition. Her skin was expressing the internal state of a nervous system under chronic stress from social deprivation. No supplement addresses that. No diet change addresses that. Because the root cause wasn't nutritional.

The root cause was that her nervous system had been in threat mode for months—and no amount of zinc or good eating was going to fix that.

New friends. Laughter. Shared evenings. Real human connection.

Her cortisol dropped. Her inflammation dropped. Her skin cleared.

The power of social connection—I didn't actually know it mattered that much. But that case showed me it matters on a level I hadn't fully appreciated before.

I want to be honest about my own experience here, because I've been on the extreme end of the other problem.

I spend most of my day inside my head. Eight-plus hours of intense cognitive focus—researching, reading, writing about health. I covered this in the last chapter. What I didn't mention there is what I've noticed about the social piece.

I am so busy with "my projects" that I isolate other people sometimes.

I learned from Dr. William Davis about an *L. reuteri* yogurt culture you can make at home that can increase your oxytocin.

Of course I had to try it.

I think I might have been taking it for a week and my wife Karen said, "What has gotten into you?"

What do you mean?

"Do you realize that you want to hug me five times a day?" I didn't even realize it.

"You also are so much more interested in other people and spending more time with them." That was fascinating to me.

The microbe *L. reuteri* is a keystone microbe that comes from your mother, if you were breastfed, and is highly sensitive to antibiotics. Mine was probably wiped out long ago, but this microbe gets your body to make more oxytocin, which has some cool effects—lowering stress, increasing your sociability, helping you sleep, and much more. See the recipe in the back of the book.

Don't make the mistake I made—treating the social environment as some optional thing you will get to at some point.

Here's the honest picture of what modern social life looks like from a biological standpoint.

Hundreds of contacts. Dozens of acquaintances. A phone full of people you could theoretically reach. Social media followers numbering in the thousands for some people. Constant exposure. Constant stimulation.

And underneath all of it—a nervous system that is profoundly under-regulated.

Your nervous system doesn't care about how many friends you have. It cares about safety, closeness, and consistency. Here is what your body is actually looking for:

- **Real Depth:** This means you have enough history and trust with someone that you can completely drop your guard. You don't feel the need to perform or impress them; you can just *be*.
- **Consistency (Repetition):** Your body relaxes when it knows what to expect. When someone is consistently there for you, your brain translates that routine into a feeling of belonging. New relationships are exciting, but they also bring uncertainty. True biological peace only comes from long-term stability. The stability *is* the medicine.
- **In-Person Connection:** Your nervous system needs the full experience—hearing a real voice, seeing facial expressions, and being close enough to touch. Digital connections just don't cut it.
- **Zero Stress:** True connection means this person doesn't trigger your anxiety or stress hormones. This is huge, and most people completely overlook it.

Ultimately, your body isn't looking for a massive social network. It's looking for a few safe, predictable places to land.

Not all connection helps. Some of it actively damages you.

There are two types of people: those who support you and bring you up and then there are others who bring you down (AKA: toxic people).

A relationship with a chronic critic elevates cortisol every time you're in it. A drama-driven person keeps your nervous system in constant stress mode. A passive-aggressive partner—someone whose mood you're constantly having to read—trains your stress response to stay on permanently, because you never know what's coming.

These relationships don't just fail to deliver oxytocin. They actively block it. You cannot regulate in a relationship where your threat system is running.

And the research on this is consistent: the quality of your close relationships predicts your inflammatory markers, your immune function, your cardiovascular health, and your lifespan more reliably than almost any other variable. Better than diet in some studies. Better than exercise in others.

The longest-running study on human health and happiness—the Harvard Study of Adult Development, running since 1938, over eighty years of data—found one thing above all others that predicted who aged well and who didn't. Not wealth. Not intelligence. Not genetics. The quality of their close relationships.

One toxic relationship in your inner circle can undermine everything else you're doing for your health. That is not an emotional statement. That is a biological fact.

Reducing or removing exposure to chronically cortisol-raising relationships is a health intervention. The same way you removed engineered food from your kitchen, the same way you got the phone out of your bedroom—sometimes the right architectural move is reducing what's in the environment, not adding more.

Pick your friends and family wisely!

For a lot of people, digital social activity has completely replaced embodied contact. They're online constantly, and genuinely wonder why they feel so alone. It's not a paradox. They're receiving stimulation without regulation. It's the same pattern as ultra-processed food—high input, low nourishment.

The body knows the difference. Even when the mind has convinced itself it's getting enough.

Here's a practical problem that connects this chapter back to Chapter 1.

Most social gatherings in the modern world are built around food and alcohol. Birthday parties, family dinners, work events, celebrations—the ritual center is almost always something your food environment shouldn't contain.

And this creates a real bind. The gathering itself is good for you—the connection, the presence, the shared time. The food at the gathering is working against you.

The solution is not to avoid the gathering. The gathering is the point. The solution is to separate your participation in the social ritual from your participation in the food ritual.

Eat before you go. Bring something. Choose protein and leave the rest. Have one short answer ready for when someone notices—"I feel better this way"—and don't elaborate. Short answers close the conversation. Long answers open debates.

The people who successfully maintain their food environment long-term are not the ones with the most willpower at the table. They're the ones who made the decision before they arrived.

Here's something worth saying directly, because the cultural message on this is completely wrong.

You do not need a wide social network. You do not need to be socially active in the way modern culture defines it. You do not need a full social calendar, or a large group of friends.

Your nervous system needs three things.

One to three people you trust completely. Deep trust, frequent enough contact to maintain genuine familiarity, relationships where you don't have to perform. This is your core. One person is enough if the relationship is genuinely deep. Three is plenty. Beyond that, you're adding contacts, not connection.

A slightly wider circle of five to fifteen people you share activities or purpose with. Not intimacy—shared doing. A workout partner. A neighbor you actually talk to. A colleague you genuinely like. These relationships provide belonging through shared activity, without requiring the depth of the inner circle.

And some sense of shared purpose. Being part of something larger than your individual relationships—a community, a cause, a project, a faith tradition, a regular group of some kind. The sense of being part of something that continues whether you show up or not is a different kind of biological input than individual relationships provide.

Beyond that, more is not better. A hundred shallow connections do not add up to one deep one. The nervous system doesn't average them. It responds to the depth and repetition of the highest-quality inputs.

The Town That Ate Lard—and Beat Heart Disease Anyway

If you think this is all theory, let me tell you about a town in Pennsylvania called Roseto.

Back in the 1950s, some researchers got curious about it. The people there were Italian immigrants, and on paper they were doing everything wrong. They cooked with lard. They ate sausage and hard cheese and bread. Plenty of them smoked. Almost none of them exercised the way we mean it today.

And they almost never had heart attacks.

The towns right next door—same water supply, same hospital, same doctors—had heart disease at the normal American rate. Roseto had a small fraction of it. The men especially. So the researchers went looking for the reason. A gene. Something in the water. They came up empty.

The reason was the town itself.

Roseto lived close. Three generations under one roof. Neighbors who knew your name and your troubles. Church, clubs, festivals, front porches. Nobody ate alone. Nobody aged alone. If something went wrong in your life, half the street knew by dinner—and showed up.

Then the next generation grew up, moved into their own houses, chased the bigger paycheck, stopped going to the clubs.

The town became like every other town. The close ties came apart.

And the heart disease arrived right on schedule. Roseto's rates climbed until they matched the neighbors they'd been beating for decades.

Sit with what that means. The diet didn't save them—they ate lard the whole way through. There were no gym memberships to thank. What protected their hearts was each other. And the moment that loosened, the protection left with it.

Boy, that one gets me every time. Because it says the thing the supplement aisle never will: connection isn't extra. Your body needs it the way it needs food. Take it away, and something starts to break—even when everything else looks perfect on paper.

What to Actually Do

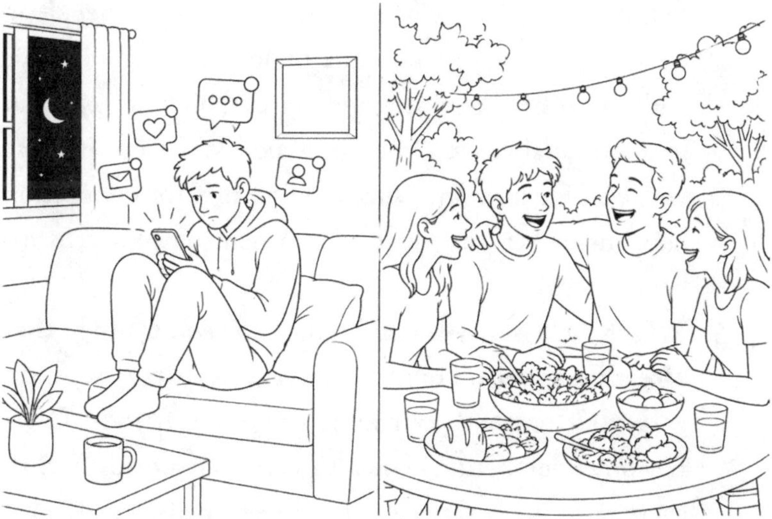

So here's where to start.

1. **Audit your inner circle first.** Who are the one to three people you feel genuinely at ease with—not performing, not managing, just present? If you can't name them, that's the most important information in this chapter. That's the gap. Not more connections—deeper ones.
2. **Identify who's raising your cortisol.** One or two names will come to mind immediately. You don't necessarily have to remove them entirely—some relationships are complicated. But be honest about whether they belong at the center of your social architecture, or whether reducing their access is a health decision, not just a personal one.
3. **Make one shared meal a standing fixture.** Don't leave it to "we should get together sometime." Put it on repeat—the same night each week, the same people, a basket by the door where the phones go. Shared meals without distraction are one of the highest oxytocin inputs available, and they cost no extra time because you're eating anyway. Once it's a fixture, the connection happens on schedule instead of when someone remembers to organize it.
4. **Attach a twenty-second hug to something that already happens.** Hugs that last at least twenty seconds, with your partner, your kids, your close friends. Don't rely on remembering—tie it to a cue that already occurs: every greeting, every goodbye, every bedtime. Then it

runs on its own. This is not sentimental advice—twenty seconds is the threshold for meaningful oxytocin release. A quick three-second hug doesn't move the chemistry the same way. Twenty seconds does.

5. **Have phone-free time with the people you care about.** The phone on the table—even face down, even silent—measurably reduces the quality of the interaction. Research shows people feel less connected in conversations where a phone is just visible, even if nobody looks at it. Remove it entirely during the time that matters.
6. **Schedule recurring time with the people who make you laugh.** You can't will yourself to laugh, but you can engineer proximity to it. Laughter is one of the fastest oxytocin and endorphin triggers available—and it requires other people to work properly. So instead of waiting for it, build the standing slot: the friends, the group, the regular night that reliably produces it. It's not entertainment. It's biochemistry. The woman whose acne cleared—she was laughing until the early hours of the morning. That's not a coincidence.
7. **If you have a pet, use it deliberately.** Animal interaction is a genuine oxytocin trigger. Not a replacement for human connection—but a real supplement to it, especially on the days when human contact is limited.
8. **Set a standing walk with one person.** Same person, same cadence—a regular walk that doesn't have to be renegotiated each time. The combination of physical presence, shared activity, and an outdoor environment

stacks three regulatory inputs at once, and putting it on repeat means it actually happens. A walk with someone you trust is doing more biological work than most people realize.

The Bottom Line

Your social environment is an environment—exactly like your food environment, your light environment, your chemical environment. It either supports your biology or it degrades it. There is no neutral.

The modern version—high exposure, low depth, digitally mediated, fragmented by geography and screens—is delivering stimulation without regulation. It looks like connection. It doesn't function like it.

The proof of that is a young woman whose acne didn't respond to a single nutritional intervention—but cleared completely when she found real friends and started laughing again every night.

Your nervous system needs what human nervous systems have always needed: a small number of stable, trustworthy, physically present people. Repeated contact. Real touch. Real voices. Shared time. Genuine laughter.

That's not a high bar. But for most people living modern lives, it takes deliberate architectural choices—because the default environment is actively working against it.

Health is not a solo project. It never was.

The biology was always designed for a tribe. You just have to build one.

Your social environment sets a baseline the others run on top of. Real connection buffers stress, shapes what and how you eat, and competes directly with the screen time from Chapter 6 for the very same hours of your day.

Next chapter: The Workspace Environment. For most people, the desk is where the majority of waking hours are spent—and it inverts nearly every signal your body was built for, all at once. We'll get into what eight hours at a screen does to your eyes, your neck and posture, your nervous system, and your focus—and exactly how to redesign the workstation so the inputs your body actually needs are built into the day instead of squeezed in afterward.

CHAPTER 8

The Workspace Environment

> **► START HERE**
>
> **The one move that unlocks everything in Chapter 8:**
> Raise your main screen until the top of it sits at eye level—stack it on books, buy a $20 stand, whatever it takes—and pull it back to about an arm's length away. You spend hours locked in front of that screen, and every inch it sits too low drags your head forward and loads your neck with tens of pounds of extra force. Fix the height once and you fix the posture for every hour after, with nothing left for you to remember. Do this before anything else in this chapter. Start here.

I want to describe my average Tuesday.

I sit down at my computer around 7:00 a.m. I'm researching—biochemistry papers, health data, cross-referencing studies. Deep focus. By the time I look up, it's often 3:00 in the afternoon. Eight hours have passed and I've barely moved. My eyes hurt. My neck is tight. My lower back is reminding me it exists. And my brain—which has been running at full capacity for eight straight hours—is simultaneously exhausted and unable to stop.

Now here's the thing. I know exactly what this is doing to my body. I study this for a living. And I still do it.

That tells you something important: this is not a knowledge problem. It's an architecture problem.

The modern workspace—desk, chair, screen, keyboard, artificial light, indoor air, zero movement, continuous cognitive demand—is one of the most extreme ancestral mismatches in this entire book. It inverts nearly everything the human body was designed for, simultaneously, for eight to ten hours a day.

And most people have been doing it for decades without ever questioning whether the environment itself is the problem.

For 99.9 percent of human history, your body spent its day doing this:

Moving constantly. Seeing into the distance. Working in natural light. Changing postures—squatting, walking, lifting, carrying. Solving problems while physically moving. Resting intermittently. Being outside.

The workspace inverts every single one of those inputs at the same time.

Fixed near-focus instead of distance vision. Artificial light instead of full-spectrum sunlight. Static sitting instead of constant varied movement. Continuous abstract cognitive demand instead of intermittent physical problem-solving. Indoors instead of outside.

This is not a minor deviation from the ancestral template. This is a complete reversal of it. And the body's response—eye strain, neck pain, lower back dysfunction, afternoon brain fog, anxiety, poor sleep, metabolic slowdown, weight gain despite reasonable eating—is not malfunction. It is a logical response to an illogical environment.

Your body is not breaking down. It's adapting to the inputs it's receiving. The inputs are wrong.

Let me start with vision, because it's the most immediate damage most people feel—and the least understood.

Humans evolved primarily using distance vision. Hunting, navigating terrain, scanning horizons, watching for threats 50 to 200 meters away. The ciliary muscle—which controls the shape of the lens—was designed to spend most of its time relaxed, in the configuration for distance viewing.

Computer work locks that muscle in continuous contraction for sustained near-focus at 30 to 70 centimeters. Hour after hour. Day after day.

And what happens to any muscle held in continuous contraction without release? It fatigues. It shortens. It loses flexibility. The ciliary muscle is no different. Over time, the lens loses accommodative range—the ability to shift fluidly between near and far. This is not genetic degeneration. It's neuromuscular conditioning. The eye is adapting to the only demand being placed on it.

Here's what most people don't know: A lot of what looks like vision decline is actually functional first. Muscle tension, neural signaling patterns, focus habits—not structural damage. And that matters, because functional adaptation can often be reversed if you catch it early enough, before the structural changes set in.

There's also this: Your blink rate drops from fifteen to

twenty blinks per minute normally to five to seven blinks per minute at a screen. That's less than half. The tear film that protects and lubricates your cornea evaporates three times faster than it's being replenished. Dry eyes, light sensitivity, corneal irritation—those aren't random. They're the direct result of a blink rate the screen is suppressing.

And then there's the light itself. Screen light is LED-dominant, blue-heavy, with no infrared, no UV, no spectral variation. Your retina one of the most metabolically active tissues in your entire body—is designed for full-spectrum sunlight that shifts through the day. Artificial screen light is nutritionally deficient light. It delivers the stimulating frequencies and none of the restorative ones. Retinal mitochondrial stress, oxidative damage, and circadian disruption all follow.

Now here's the connection most people miss: Vision is not just a mechanical process. It's a neurological one.

The eye delivers signals. The brain interprets them. And the quality of that interpretation depends heavily on your nervous system state. When you're stressed, fatigued, or in sympathetic overdrive—which is exactly what sustained computer work produces—visual processing degrades. The clarity fluctuates with your stress level, not just with your lens prescription.

And this is why staring is a problem beyond just ciliary muscle fatigue. Fixed gaze is a threat-physiology response. Your eyes evolved to stare when something dangerous was in front of you. Fixed gaze narrows your peripheral vision, activates the sympathetic nervous system, suppresses blinking, and increases tension in the neck and jaw. So staring at a screen for hours is running a low-grade threat response continuously. Your nervous system cannot tell the difference between staring at a predator and staring at a spreadsheet.

Boy, when I first understood that connection—that my eye strain was partly a stress response, not just a focus problem—it changed how I thought about the whole thing.

So what do you actually do about your eyes? The principle is simple: Whatever the screen takes away, you give back. The screen locks your focus at one distance, so you deliberately send it long. The screen suppresses your blink, so you blink on purpose. The screen feeds you one narrow band of artificial light, so you go get the real thing.

The core move is the near-far reset. Every twenty to thirty minutes, look up and find the farthest thing you can—out a window, down a hallway, across the room—and hold it for at least twenty seconds. Some people know this as the 20-20-20 rule: every 20 minutes, look 20 feet away, for 20 seconds. Whatever you call it, what it does is let the ciliary muscle release the contraction it has been holding. The best version is real distance outdoors, because nothing indoors is truly far—and the natural light is doing a second job for your retina at the same time.

Then there's blinking, which sounds too simple to matter and isn't. At a screen, your blink rate drops by more than half, and the blinks you do manage are often incomplete. So every few minutes, do one slow, full blink—all the way closed, all the way open. And once or twice a day, try palming: rub your hands together until they're warm, cup them gently over your closed eyes without pressing, and sit in that warm darkness for a minute. It relaxes the eye muscles and gives the visual system a genuine rest from light input—a small thing that feels surprisingly good after a long screen day.

And get your eyes outside. The same morning light that sets your clock back in Chapter 2 is also the richest visual environment your eyes ever get—full-spectrum, full of depth, full of real distance. Fifteen minutes of looking at the actual world, shifting focus near and far, near and far, is physical therapy for a visual system that spends all day frozen at arm's length. The eyes run on a muscle system like anything else. Lock them in one position all day and they stiffen. Give them range, and a surprising amount of what looks like permanent decline turns out to be reversible.

Here's the mainstream position on sitting: it's not ideal, but as long as you exercise, you're fine.

That is so not true.

An hour at the gym does not cancel eight hours of sitting. I said this in Chapter 3, and I want to say it again here, because it's the most important thing in this chapter that most people reject.

Sitting doesn't just weaken muscles. It turns off metabolic processes that are only activated by muscle contraction. Lipoprotein lipase—critical for fat metabolism—drops within hours of continuous sitting. Glucose uptake into muscle tissue slows. Insulin sensitivity degrades. Circulation to the lower body reduces significantly.

These are not effects a morning workout reverses. They

accumulate across the hours of sitting, regardless of what you did at 6:00 a.m.

Immobility is not neutral. Prolonged stillness is an active signal to the body: downshift circulation, downshift glucose metabolism, downshift repair. The body interprets sustained inactivity as a physiological instruction. And it follows that instruction whether you intend it to or not.

The structural damage is just as significant. Chair sitting was not part of human evolution. Ancestral rest postures—squatting, ground sitting with frequent transitions, kneeling—maintained hip mobility, spinal load distribution, and pelvic alignment. Chair sitting shortens the hip flexors, inhibits the glutes, compresses the lumbar discs, and reduces spinal fluid dynamics. Over years, this produces the pattern most desk workers know well: lower back pain, tight hips, a pelvis that doesn't move correctly, and a spine that has structurally adapted to one position.

The head-forward posture that screens produce is its own problem. For every inch your head moves forward from neutral, the effective load on your cervical spine increases by roughly ten pounds. Most people working at a screen have their head displaced two to three inches forward. That's twenty to thirty additional pounds of load on a structure that wasn't designed for it—eight hours a day, five days a week, for decades.

That's not a posture problem. That's a structural engineering problem.

And there's a detail here almost nobody talks about: The vagus nerve—the primary pathway of the parasympathetic nervous system—passes through the neck. Chronic upper cervical tension from forward head posture physically impairs vagal signaling. This is one of the reasons desk workers so often have digestive issues, difficulty relaxing, and a nervous system that never fully comes down. The mechanical compression is affecting the nerve that runs the entire recovery system.

So, if sitting bends you into a shape—hips closed, chest collapsed, head jutting forward—the antidote is to spend a little time each day bending the other way. Not a workout. Just a handful of positions that reverse the exact compressions the desk creates. Tie them to the movement break you're already taking every forty-five to sixty minutes, and they cost you almost nothing.

Open the hip flexors. These are the muscles that shorten from hours of sitting, and short hip flexors are a major driver of the lower-back pain desk workers live with. Drop into a half-kneeling lunge—one knee down, the other foot planted in front—and gently push your hips forward until you feel the stretch down the front of the back leg. Thirty seconds each side. If you do one stretch in this whole chapter, do this one.

Open the chest and upper back. Sitting rounds you forward; you counter it by extending back. Stand in a doorway, forearms on the frame, and lean through to stretch across the chest. Or sit tall, lace your hands behind your head, and arch gently back over the top of your chair to extend the part of your spine that's been slumped all day. This is the direct antidote to the rounded, collapsed posture the screen builds into you.

Decompress the neck. For the forward-head load we just

talked about, the fix is the chin tuck—not dropping your chin, but sliding your whole head straight back over your shoulders, like making a double chin on purpose. Hold it five seconds; repeat several times. It re-stacks your head over your spine and takes the strain off the structures—and the vagus nerve—running through your neck. A slow shoulder roll and a gentle ear-to-shoulder stretch on each side finish the job.

Wake the glutes and move the spine. Sitting switches the glutes off; a few standing hip bridges—or even just standing and squeezing them hard for ten seconds—reminds them they have a job. Then move your spine through its range: a slow cat-cow, rounding and arching, or a few gentle standing back-bends and side-bends. The spine is built to move in every direction. A chair only ever lets it do one.

None of this takes more than two or three minutes. The point isn't a stretching routine you'll abandon by Thursday. It's a few targeted positions, attached to a break you're already taking, that undo the specific shape the desk is pressing into you—before it sets.

Here's the mismatch that's invisible, because it doesn't produce a physical symptom you can point to.

For most of human evolution, thinking was situational, intermittent, and paired with physical movement. You solved problems while walking, tracking, building, working with your hands. Abstract reasoning existed—humans are problem-solvers—but it was brief, contextual, and followed by physical resolution.

Computer work requires something that has never existed

before: sustained abstract reasoning for eight to ten hours, completely uncoupled from physical movement, in a low-sensory environment, with continuous decision-making and no natural endpoints.

The prefrontal cortex—which handles logic, planning, error correction, and inhibition—was designed for short bursts, not continuous operation. When you push it past ninety minutes without a genuine break, performance degrades. Creativity drops. Decision quality falls. Irritability rises. This is not weakness—it's a hardware limitation being exceeded.

The neurotransmitter side is just as real. Sustained focus depletes dopamine, acetylcholine, and norepinephrine—the chemical substrates of motivation, focus, and alertness. When they drop, the brain sends a signal most people misread: reach for caffeine, reach for food, reach for stimulation. It's not hunger. It's neurochemical depletion. The snacking, the coffee, the compulsive phone-checking that happens around two or three in the afternoon—that's your depleted brain trying to find fuel.

And then there's the cortisol problem. Problem-solving stress elevates cortisol. In ancestral conditions, cortisol was paired with movement—the physical activity metabolized the stress hormones and brought the system back down. At a computer, cortisol rises from cognitive stress and has nowhere to go. No physical discharge. It stays elevated, builds through the afternoon, degrades your sleep quality that night, and starts the next day already elevated.

This is what burnout actually is at the biological level. It's not overwork in the abstract. It's the accumulation of undischarged cortisol from cognitive stress that was never paired with the physical release the body expected.

Now, I want to be honest here, because I live at the extreme end of this problem.

Eight-plus hours of cognitive hyperfocus daily. This is my actual life. I'm not describing someone else's situation—I'm describing mine.

Here's what I've figured out through trial and error, a lot of it painful.

The two hours I spend outside every day without my phone—which I talked about in Chapter 6—are not a luxury. They are non-negotiable biological infrastructure. Without them, the cognitive load of the morning builds past the point of recovery, and the next day starts already compromised. With them, I can sustain the deep focus work for years without burning out.

But I've also had to accept something that took me longer than it should have to admit: I cannot out-supplement a bad work environment. I know exactly which nutrients support cognitive function—DHA, magnesium, B vitamins, choline. I take them. They help. But if I don't move, if I don't get outside, if I don't break the screen exposure and the near-focus lock and the continuous cognitive demand—the supplements do maybe 20 percent of the job. The environment does the other 80 percent.

The physical architecture of my workspace matters. The breaks matter. The outdoor time matters. The movement matters. The eye resets matter. Not as nice-to-haves—as the primary intervention, with nutrition supporting it.

Don't make the mistake I made for years, thinking you can compensate your way out of a bad environment with the right supplement protocol. You can't. Fix the environment first. Then the supplements do what they're supposed to do.

I addressed EMF back in Chapter 4, and I want to bring it back here specifically in the context of the workspace—because the computer environment stacks the exposure in a way the home environment alone doesn't.

Wi-Fi router. Bluetooth keyboard, mouse, and headphones. Phone on the desk or in your pocket. Laptop power supply. Multiple screens and charging cables. In a typical workspace, you're sitting inside a cluster of continuously transmitting devices for eight hours a day.

And remember what I said about EMF in Chapter 4: the concern is not intensity. It's duration. Brief high-intensity exposure is not the same biological stressor as continuous, low-level exposure across eight hours. It's the duration that does the damage, not the intensity.

So a few simple structural rules—they cost nothing, and require no special equipment.

Don't put your laptop on your lap. Ever. Use a desk or a hard barrier. The heat alone is a problem, and the proximity to your reproductive tissue and abdomen during hours of daily use is unnecessary exposure that's trivially easy to avoid.

Don't keep your phone in your pocket during work. Put it on the desk, away from your body. The device is transmitting continuously whether you're using it or not.

Prefer wired Internet at a fixed desk. Not always practical—but when it is, a wired Ethernet connection eliminates the Wi-Fi exposure from your immediate environment entirely.

And increase your distance from the router and the power bricks. Distance matters more than any shielding product. Two feet of additional distance produces a dramatic reduction in field intensity. You don't need gadgets. You need geometry.

A few more, just as easy. Turn off the radios you're not using—Bluetooth and Wi-Fi on a device that's plugged into Ethernet are transmitting for no reason. When you're not expecting calls, airplane mode is the simplest off switch there is. And when you do take a call on your cell, don't hold it against your head—use speakerphone, wired earbuds, or an air-tube headset, and keep the phone off your body. Holding a transmitting phone to your skull is the highest-intensity exposure most people get all day, and it's completely avoidable.

One more thing worth knowing: A phone works hardest when the signal is weakest. In a basement, an elevator, a moving car, anywhere the bars are low, the phone cranks up its transmitting power to stay connected—so that's the worst time to hold it close. If the signal is bad and the call isn't urgent, text instead, or wait until you've got a strong signal. Little choices, made daily, that lower the duration of close-range exposure—which, remember, is the whole game with EMF.

And at night—which I've said twice now, but it bears repeating—phone out of the bedroom, Wi-Fi off if you can, no charging devices next to your head. The bedroom is your primary recovery environment. It should be the one place in your life that has genuine signal silence.

What to Actually Do

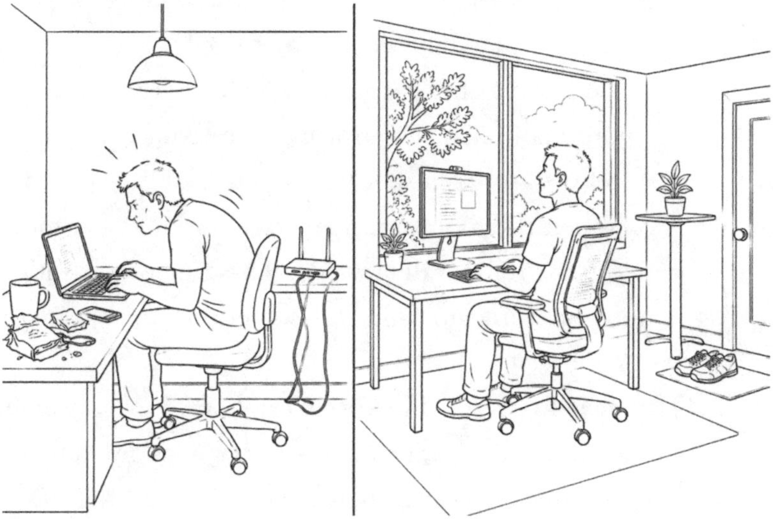

Here's the honest priority order—not everything at once, but in the order of what moves the needle most.

1. **The forty-five-minute rule.** Every forty-five to sixty minutes at the desk, you get up and move for at least five minutes. Not stretching in your chair. Not standing at a standing desk. Actually moving through space—walking down a hallway, going outside briefly, doing something that changes your joint angles and reloads your muscles. Set a timer. Don't rely on memory. This one rule, applied consistently, changes the metabolic picture of the entire work day.
2. **Build two or three work positions into the room.** A standing desk is not the answer to a sitting

problem—static standing for eight hours is not meaningfully better than static sitting. What matters is position variety, and the reliable way to get it is to build it into the space rather than try to remember to shift. Set up more than one place to work: a seated desk, a raised surface to stand at, a spot where you take calls on your feet. When the room offers several positions, you move between them naturally instead of holding one. Position is not something to hold. It's something to repeatedly reset.

3. **The near-far reset, hourly.** Every hour, look at something as far away as possible—out a window, down a hallway, outside—and then back to something close. Alternate five to ten times. The way to make this automatic is to point your desk at a window, so the far target and the natural light are always right there instead of something you have to go find. This is the single most effective thing you can do for ciliary muscle flexibility. It takes sixty seconds. Do it every time the forty-five-minute timer goes off.
4. **Blink deliberately.** Every few minutes at a screen, do a slow, full blink. Not a rapid flutter—a slow, complete closure and reopening. This re-wets the tear film and partially counteracts the blink suppression the screen produces. Simple. Free. It works.
5. **Fix your screen position.** The top of your monitor should be at or slightly below eye level. If you're on a laptop at a desk, you need a stand and a separate keyboard—laptop

height forces a chronic neck flexion that is a structural injury happening in slow motion. This is a one-time fix with permanent benefit.

6. **Apply the workspace EMF rules.** Laptop never on your lap—desk or hard barrier only. Phone off your body and on the desk, not in your pocket. Wired internet over Wi-Fi when it's practical. Two extra feet of distance from your router and power bricks. Turn off Bluetooth and Wi-Fi on anything that's already wired in. These cost nothing and require no equipment—just geometry and habit.
7. **Stretch the desk out of you.** At your movement breaks, run through a few targeted positions that reverse the desk shape—a half-kneeling hip-flexor lunge, a doorway or behind-the-head chest opener, and a chin tuck to re-stack your head over your spine. Two or three minutes, tied to a break you're already taking. This undoes the specific compressions sitting builds in, before they set into permanent posture.
8. **Cap your deep work blocks at ninety minutes.** The brain evolved for intermittent load. After ninety minutes, take a genuine break—outside if possible, away from screens, with movement. Not a coffee refill. A real break that lets the prefrontal cortex recover.
9. **Make a walk the built-in exit from deep work.** When you finish an intense cognitive session, don't go straight to your phone or a video. Set it up so the walk is the path of least resistance—shoes by the office door, the screen

not the nearest thing to reach for. Walk first, move first, and give the cortisol that built during the session a physical outlet before you introduce more stimulation. This is the difference between ending the workday recovered versus ending it wired and depleted.

10. **Use the nutrients that support the cognitive load.** DHA first—the structural fat of neuronal membranes; it reduces neuroinflammation and improves signal efficiency. Magnesium second—it calms neuronal firing, reduces excitotoxicity, and supports sleep after mental work. B vitamins third—essential for neurotransmitter synthesis and glucose metabolism in the brain. These don't replace the environmental fixes. They support the biology the environmental fixes are trying to protect.
11. **Anchor one outdoor break to a cue that already happens.** Not at your desk by a window—outside. Tie it to something fixed in the day so it doesn't get skipped: lunch eaten outdoors, a standing midday walk, the first thing after your hardest block. Natural light, distance vision, fresh air. Even ten minutes resets the visual system, delivers the light signal your circadian clock needs, and provides a genuine nervous system state change that no indoor break replicates.

The Bottom Line

The workspace is the environment where most people spend the majority of their waking hours. And for most people, it is simultaneously degrading their vision, their posture, their metabolism, their nervous system, their sleep, and their cognitive capacity—every day, compounding over years.

None of those things are inevitable. They're the result of a specific environment that was designed for productivity, without any consideration of biology.

The fix is not a standing desk or a blue light filter. Those are downstream patches on an upstream architecture problem. The fix is redesigning the environment so that the inputs the body actually requires—movement, varied vision, natural light, intermittent cognitive demand, nervous system recovery—are built into the workday by default, rather than squeezed in as afterthoughts.

I do eight-plus hours of deep cognitive work every day. And I intend to keep doing it for a long time. The only way I've found to make that sustainable is to treat the workspace as an environment to be designed—not just a place to show up.

The biology is non-negotiable. Work with it, or work against it. The results are very different.

The workspace is where several environments collide at once: the sitting from Chapter 3, the screen light and eye strain tied to Chapter 2, and the fractured attention from Chapter 6. Redesign the desk well and you move all three at the same time.

Next chapter: The Nutrient Infrastructure. You can fix every environment in this book and still run below capacity if the raw materials aren't there. The modern food supply has been quietly stripped of the vitamins, minerals, and cofactors your biology runs on—so you can be overfed and undernourished at the same time. We'll get into exactly where the gaps are, why they matter, and how to close them with food first and a short, specific supplement list second.

CHAPTER 9

The Nutrient Infrastructure

► **START HERE**

The one move that unlocks everything in Chapter 9:

Get your vitamin D level tested—then take vitamin D3 with K2 at the fattiest meal of your day. Vitamin D is the one nutrient where a simple blood test gives you genuinely actionable numbers, and low D is among the most common and most correctable shortfalls of a modern indoor life. Test first so you're closing a real gap instead of guessing; then attach the D3-with-K2 to a meal you already eat so it becomes automatic. Start here.

Here's a sentence that should not be possible in the wealthiest country in human history:

You can be overfed and starving at the same time.

Not starving for calories. Starving for the raw materials your body needs to actually function—the vitamins, minerals, trace elements, and cofactors that run every enzymatic reaction, every mitochondrial process, every repair pathway, every hormonal signal in your body.

And this is happening to most people eating what they consider a reasonable diet. Not because they're eating too little. Because the food supply has been quietly stripped of the things that matter most—and nobody told them.

In Chapter 1 we covered how the food environment sends the wrong signals to your metabolism. That's a distortion problem. This chapter is different. This is a capacity problem.

Think of it this way. Chapter 1 was about corrupted software—the instructions going into the system are wrong. This chapter is about missing hardware—the machinery required to run any instructions at all isn't there.

You can treat the symptoms perfectly. You can time your meals correctly. You can eliminate seed oils and eat real food and close the kitchen at 7:00 p.m. And your metabolism will still underperform if the cofactors aren't there.

Cofactors: vitamins and minerals that biochemical reactions depend upon.

Because without the cofactors, the enzymes don't work. And without the enzymes, nothing works—not completely, not efficiently, not long-term.

This is the silent layer. And it's the one most people never find.

Your great-grandparents didn't take supplements. And they also didn't need to—not most of them, not systematically. Not because they were nutritionally perfect, but because the food infrastructure around them delivered a nutrient density the modern food supply no longer provides by default.

Here's what that infrastructure looked like. Mineral-rich soil that hadn't been depleted by decades of monocrop agriculture. Animals that grazed on diverse pasture and ate what they evolved to eat. Whole-animal (nose to tail) eating—not just muscle meat, but organs, bone marrow, connective tissue, collagen-rich cuts. Water that carried dissolved minerals from the ground it traveled through. Seafood eaten regularly, in coastal and inland communities alike. Seasonal vegetables grown in genuinely fertile soil.

And every one of those inputs has been systematically degraded or removed.

The soil is depleted. Repeated monocropping (growing just one thing) without mineral replenishment has stripped the trace elements out of agricultural land across most of the developed world. The food grown in that soil contains less magnesium, less zinc, less selenium, less copper than the same food grown fifty years ago. And this isn't controversial—it's documented in USDA nutritional data going back to the 1950s. The same apple. Measurably less nutrition.

The animals are grain-fed, confined, and nutrient-altered. A grass-fed animal eating diverse pasture has a fundamentally different nutritional profile than a grain-fed animal in a concentrated feeding operation. Different fatty acid ratios. Different fat-soluble vitamin content. Different micronutrient density. On my farm, the cows and other animals consume a lot of weeds with the grasses, giving them a wide variety of plant-based compounds (polyphenols), which help build up antioxidants in the meat.

The nose-to-tail eating is gone. Every traditional food culture on Earth ate the whole animal—liver, kidney, heart, brain, marrow, connective tissue, skin, bone broth. These parts contain nutrients that muscle meat simply doesn't provide. Real vitamin A—retinol, not the beta-carotene precursor—lives in liver. Copper lives in liver. CoQ10 lives in heart. Glycine lives in connective tissue and bone broth. K2 lives in certain organ meats and fermented foods. The modern grocery store sells you the muscle and throws away the nutrition.

The water is stripped. Reverse osmosis systems, heavy municipal filtration, bottled demineralized water these deliver hydration without minerals. Water traveling through rock and soil used to be a meaningful source of magnesium, calcium, and trace elements. Back in the day our magnesium source came from spring water. Now we soften the water and remove it.

The result of all this together is what I call a mineral collapse architecture. The food exists. The calories are there. But the cofactor (nutrient) density—the actual fuel for the biological machinery—has been quietly engineered out of the default food supply.

Let me explain why this matters so much, because "vitamins and minerals are important" is advice people have been ignoring for decades. And the reason it gets ignored is that nobody explains the mechanism clearly enough to make it feel urgent.

So here's the mechanism.

Almost everything your body does is run by tiny worker proteins called enzymes. Think of them as the machines on a factory floor—they do the actual work. But here's the catch: Most of these machines won't switch on until a specific part is snapped into place. And that part is a mineral or a vitamin. No part, no work. That little part has a name—a cofactor—and it physically plugs into the enzyme and turns it on.

Magnesium is required for over three hundred enzymatic reactions. Not helpful for three hundred reactions. Required. Without it, those reactions either don't happen, or they happen at severely reduced efficiency. ATP—the energy currency your cells run on—has to be bound to magnesium to even be biologically active. So without adequate magnesium, your energy production is structurally compromised at the cellular level, regardless of how well you eat otherwise.

Zinc is required for over two hundred enzymatic reactions. Immune function, wound healing, protein synthesis, DNA repair, testosterone production—all of it needs zinc as a physical component of the enzymes doing the work.

B vitamins are what I call the metabolic ignition keys. Thiamine—B1—is what turns the carbohydrates you eat into usable energy. Without enough of it, you can eat all the food you want and your cells still can't pull the energy out of it. B12 builds the insulation that wraps around your nerves, so the signals travel cleanly. Folate is needed to build and copy DNA every time one of your cells divides. Every B vitamin has its own specific job, and nothing else can fill in for it.

Iodine is required for thyroid hormone synthesis. Not helpful for it. Required. Without iodine, the thyroid cannot make T3 and T4—and thyroid hormones regulate the metabolic rate in virtually every cell in your body. Iodine deficiency doesn't produce dramatic symptoms right away. It produces a slow metabolic depression that looks like a dozen other problems.

Selenium runs one of your main antioxidant tools—part of the crew that mops up cellular damage before it piles up.

Without selenium, that tool is missing a piece. It's there, but it can't do the job. So your defenses run weak no matter how many antioxidant foods you eat.

This is the invisible layer. You can't feel a selenium deficiency the way you feel a broken leg. You feel it as low resilience, poor recovery, reduced stress tolerance, and a metabolism that just doesn't perform the way it should. The symptoms are diffuse, non-specific, and easily blamed on a dozen other things.

Which is exactly why it goes unfixed for years.

And here's the part that makes this problem self-perpetuating once it starts.

Micronutrient depletion lowers your stress tolerance. Lower stress tolerance means your stress system switches on more easily—more cortisol, more of that wired, on-edge feeling. Chronic stress then burns through magnesium, B vitamins, and vitamin C even faster—torching what little reserve you have. Which depletes you further. Which drops your stress tolerance lower still.

Stress doesn't cause the depletion. The depletion makes stress intolerable. And then the stress accelerates the depletion. Round and round.

This is why people can do everything right—clean diet, regular exercise, reasonable sleep—and still feel like they're running on empty.

There's also a genetic piece worth knowing about, and I'll keep it simple. Some people are just born needing more of certain nutrients than other people. You may have heard of one called MTHFR—it's common, and don't get hung up on the name. Here's all it means: The folate and B12 in your food have to be converted into a form your body can actually use, and this gene makes that conversion slow. So you need more of the "active" forms—the ones that come already converted, ready to go—to get the same result everyone else gets. There are other genes that do similar things with other nutrients.

Your genes don't cause the shortage—the food supply does that. But if you were born needing more, and the food supply is handing you less, the gap opens up faster for you than for the person sitting right next to you eating the exact same meals.

Let me be specific, because "eat more nutrients" is not useful advice. Here's exactly where the gaps are.

Fat-soluble vitamins: A, D, E, K2. These need fat to absorb, and they're found primarily in animal fat, organ meats, and full-fat dairy. The low-fat dietary movement of the last fifty years removed the primary delivery vehicles for these vitamins from the default diet. Vitamin D deficiency now affects an estimated 40 percent of American adults—get more sun exposure. Real vitamin A—retinol, not beta-carotene—is found almost exclusively in liver, full-fat dairy, and egg yolks. If you're not eating those, you're probably not getting it.

B vitamins. Depleted by refined-carbohydrate diets, alcohol, chronic stress, antibiotics, proton pump inhibitors, and oral contraceptives. B1 specifically gets depleted by sugar metabolism—every gram of refined carbohydrate you process burns through thiamine. So high-carbohydrate modern diets are burning B vitamins at a rate the depleted food supply can't replenish.

Magnesium. This one deserves its own emphasis. Soil depletion has reduced the magnesium content in food crops significantly. Stress burns it continuously. Insulin resistance impairs its retention. The kidneys excrete more of it under stress and with diuretic use. An estimated 50 to 60 percent of Americans are below the recommended daily intake—and the recommended intake is itself probably set too low. Magnesium deficiency alone can produce anxiety, muscle cramps, constipation, insomnia, insulin resistance, and cardiac arrhythmia. Boy—all of those, from one missing mineral.

Trace minerals: zinc, selenium, iodine, copper, chromium. These come from seafood, organ meats, and mineral-rich soil. So modern diets that are low in seafood, devoid of organ meats, and grown on depleted soil are structurally deficient in this entire category. Iodine was partially addressed by iodized salt—but as people cut back on table salt and shift to sea salt or pink salt, which isn't meaningfully iodized, even that partial solution disappears.

Electrolytes: potassium, sodium, chloride. The low-salt health messaging of recent decades produced a widespread fear of sodium without addressing the real issue—which is that potassium, not sodium, is the electrolyte most people are dramatically deficient in. Ancestral diets delivered an estimated 4,700 milligrams of potassium a day. The average

American gets around 2,500. That gap affects blood pressure, fluid balance, muscle function, and stress hormone regulation every single day.

Glycine and the collagen amino acids. The modern protein culture—protein powders, chicken breast, lean cuts—gives you plenty of the muscle-building amino acids and almost none of the glycine and the other building blocks found in connective tissue. Those are what your body uses to repair joints, rebuild the gut lining, and make glutathione, its master antioxidant and cleanup molecule. Run short on glycine, and the detox pathway we covered in Chapter 4 can't run at full power, no matter what else you do.

And mineral-depleted water. A subtle one, but real. Water that's passed through mineral-rich geology used to provide meaningful daily magnesium and calcium. Reverse osmosis, water softening, and heavy filtration remove that. If your drinking water is RO-filtered—which is excellent for taking out contaminants—you need to re-mineralize it. A pinch of a good sea salt, or a mineral concentrate, does it. Don't strip the minerals out and replace them with nothing.

Now, I want to be direct about this, because the supplement industry has turned nutrient support into a complicated, expensive, anxiety-producing enterprise. It does not need to be.

Here's my list—not a protocol, not a product recommendation, just what I've found actually moves the needle, based on years of research and personal use.

Magnesium. Every day. This is the one I'd keep if I could only keep one. The modern environment depletes it through stress, through the food supply, through sweat. Most people are low. And the effects of correcting it are usually noticeable within a week—better sleep, less muscle tension, less anxiety, better bowel regularity. The gold standard is magnesium glycinate because of its high absorption and bowel tolerance.

Vitamin D with K2. Unless you're outside in direct sunlight for extended periods regularly—which most people are not—you're almost certainly running low. The K2 matters here because it directs the calcium that vitamin D mobilizes into bone and arterial tissue, where it belongs, rather than into soft tissue, where it doesn't. Based on all the barriers to absorption, 10,000 IU a day with 100 mcg of K2 might be a good dose to shoot for.

Omega-3. Specifically DHA and EPA, from fish oil or algae. The omega-6 to omega-3 ratio in the modern diet runs 15 to 20 to 1. The ancestral ratio was closer to 4 to 1. Correcting that ratio reduces systemic inflammation across every system in the body. Cod liver oil has both omega-3 and vitamin D and A.

B vitamins. A B-complex in the "active" forms. On the label, that means methylfolate instead of folic acid, and hydroxocobalamin instead of cyanocobalamin. Fancy words, but all they mean is "already converted and ready for your body to use"—so they work even if you're one of the people who are slow at doing that conversion. You don't need to understand the chemistry. Just look for "active" or "methylated" on the bottle.

Iodine. Underappreciated. Underconsumed. The thyroid requires it, and most people eating a modern diet without regular seafood or seaweed are running below optimal. Start low and go slow—iodine supplementation needs gradual introduction, especially if you've been deficient for a long time. There is also a lot of additional trace minerals that are hard to get: zinc, copper, selenium, magnesium, etc. So finding a high-quality trace mineral product could handle all at once.

That's the core list. Not thirty supplements. Five or six, taken consistently, chosen for specific mechanistic reasons, attached to a fixed daily routine so they actually get taken.

The mistake I see constantly—and that I made myself early on—is reactive supplement stacking. You read about something, you add it. You hear about something else, you add that. Within a few months you've got twenty supplements and no idea which ones are working.

And I want to close this part with something I feel strongly about.

Supplements support. They don't restore.

You cannot supplement your way out of a food environment that delivers no real nutrient density. Pills don't replace organ meats. Capsules don't replace mineral-rich real food. A multivitamin is not a substitute for a diet that delivers the cofactors in their bioavailable, food-matrix form.

The right order is this. Fix the food first. Build your meals around nutrient-dense anchors—eggs with the yolks, red meat, fatty fish, leafy greens, whole-food fats. Add organ meat once a week—liver specifically. Eat bone broth or collagen-rich cuts regularly. Add mineralized water. And grow the variety of plant foods to at least twenty to thirty different ones a week.

Then use supplements to fill the specific gaps the food environment can't close—primarily D3, magnesium, omega-3, trace minerals, and B vitamins, for most people.

In that order. Not the other way around.

What to Actually Do

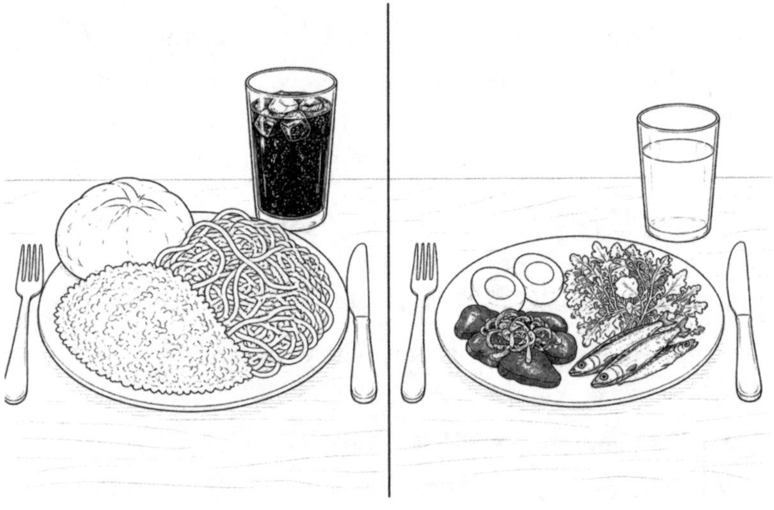

Here's the build—food first, then the gaps. And none of it runs on memory or willpower: the move is to stock these things so they're already in the house, and anchor each one to a cue or a place—a fixed night, a specific meal, the bedside—so it happens by default instead of depending on you to remember.

1. **Keep liver in the freezer and pick a night for it.** This is the single highest-return food addition most people can make—beef liver has more bioavailable vitamin A, B12, copper, zinc, and folate per gram than any other food. The reason people don't eat it is friction, so remove it: keep portions in the freezer and give it a standing slot, the same night each week. Cook it with onions and butter. One serving a week. That's it.
2. **Eat eggs with the yolks daily, if you're not already.** The yolk is where the nutrition lives—choline, lutein, real vitamin A precursors, B vitamins, selenium, iodine. The egg white on its own is a protein delivery system with most of the micronutrients stripped out.
3. **Keep a stack of tinned sardines in the pantry.** Fatty fish at least twice a week, and sardines are the most nutrient-dense and least contaminated option—they cover omega-3, iodine, selenium, D3, and B12 simultaneously, in one food. Tinned, they keep for years and need no cooking, so a stocked shelf turns "twice a week" into a no-effort default. Salmon, mackerel, and anchovies count too.
4. **Add bone broth or collagen-rich cuts weekly.** This closes the glycine gap directly, and supports gut-lining integrity, joint health, and glutathione production all at once.

5. **Re-mineralize your filtered water.** If you use RO filtration—which you should, for contaminant removal—add a pinch of a good mineral-rich sea salt, or a liquid mineral concentrate, to your drinking water. Don't strip the minerals out and replace them with nothing.
6. **Eat a large green salad daily.** Potassium, magnesium, folate, vitamin K1, fiber for the microbiome. This is the primary delivery vehicle for the electrolyte and B vitamin density most people are missing.
7. **Put the magnesium on the nightstand.** Every night—and the bottle sitting by your bed is what makes "every night" actually happen, because the cue is right where you'll be. Glycinate or malate forms absorb best and cause the least digestive disruption. Start at 200 to 400 milligrams, move up if you need to, and judge it by your sleep quality, your muscle tension, and your bowel regularity—not by lab values alone.
8. **Take D3 with K2 at your fattiest meal, in winter or if you're mostly indoors.** Attaching it to the fattiest meal isn't just a memory trick—these are fat-soluble, so they absorb far better with food that contains fat. A reasonable starting point for adults is 10,000 IU of D3 with 100 mcg of K2 (MK-7). Get your levels tested if you can—vitamin D is one of the few nutrients where testing gives you genuinely actionable data.
9. **Use a weekly pill organizer.** This is the boring little tool that makes the whole supplement list actually work. Fill it once at the start of the week, and from then on you

can see at a glance whether you've taken everything—no remembering, no guessing, no "Wait, did I already take that?" The organizer does the remembering for you, so a missed day is obvious instead of invisible. Set it where the cue already is—by the coffee for the morning ones, on the nightstand for the magnesium at night.

10. **Make the table a screen-free zone.** Eat away from the desk, with no phone or screen at the table, and take ten slow breaths before the first bite. Set the rule once so calm eating is the default, not a thing you remember. Parasympathetic dominance during eating is not a nice-to-have—it's what lets the digestive system actually extract the nutrients from the food you just paid for. Eating at a desk while answering emails is nutritionally different from eating the same food in a relaxed state. The absorption rate itself changes.

The Bottom Line

You can do everything right with your food signals, and your timing, and your sleep, and your movement—and still have a metabolism running below capacity, if the cofactors aren't there.

That's not a failure of effort. It's a failure of infrastructure. The modern food supply quietly stripped the nutrient density out of the default diet over sixty years. Most people don't know it happened. They just feel the effects—the fatigue that doesn't fully resolve, the stress tolerance that seems lower than it should be, the recovery that takes longer than it used to—without ever identifying the cause.

The cause is missing machinery. The fix is restoring the supply.

Food first. Organ meat weekly. Fatty fish twice a week. Eggs with the yolks daily. And a short, specific supplement list, chosen for mechanistic reasons and actually taken consistently.

Not complicated. Just the things the food infrastructure stopped delivering on its own.

Nutrients are the thread running through every chapter before this one—there's little point perfecting the signals if the raw materials to act on them aren't there. With all nine environments now on the table, Part Two is where they stop being nine separate fixes and start working as a single operating system.

PART II
THE OPERATING SYSTEM
Rules, Protocols, and Reference Tools

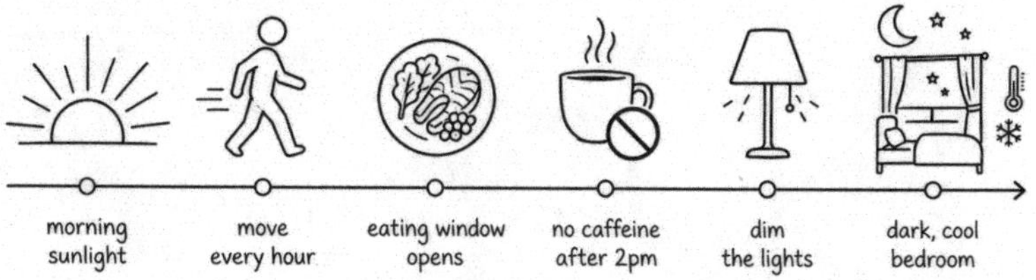

A Note Before the Rules

You've just read nine chapters about environments.

Here's the honest summary of all of it, in one paragraph:

Your body is not broken. It is responding correctly to the wrong environment. Every system we covered—food, light, sleep, movement, chemicals, microbiome, cognition, social connection, the workspace, and the nutrient infrastructure underneath all of it—is either sending your biology accurate information or inaccurate information. When the information is wrong, the biology goes wrong. Not because of weakness. Because that's how biology works.

The fix is not willpower. It's architecture.

What follows are the rules, protocols, and reference tools for building that architecture. Not one time—as a permanent operating system.

A companion for this: if you'd rather not run all of this on paper, the wellnessMAP app is built to do exactly that. It walks you through these environments one change at a time and keeps the operating system running in the background of your day.

The Master Rules

These govern every environment in the book. When in doubt, come back here.

Rule 1—Environment Before Willpower. Every Time.

Willpower is finite. It depletes through the day, and it fails when you're tired, stressed, hungry, or emotional—which is exactly when the environment is testing you most.

A well-designed environment doesn't require willpower. The right choice is just the easy choice. Design the environment first, and the willpower question becomes irrelevant. Every protocol in this section runs on this principle. If you take nothing else from this book, take this.

Rule 2—What's Visible Is What You'll Do.

What sits on your counter, you'll eat. What's at eye level in the fridge, you'll reach for first. What's on your phone's home screen, you'll open. What's charged on your nightstand, you'll check at 2:00 a.m.

Visibility is not neutral—it's a continuous behavioral trigger. Audit every environment for what's visible, then move it, hide it, or remove it. That single action, repeated across your food, digital, bedroom, and workspace, does more behavioral work than any resolution ever will.

Rule 3—Decisions Made in Advance Beat Decisions Made in the Moment.

Every single time. A person who decides what they'll order before they reach the restaurant is operating from a clear, unfatigued prefrontal cortex. A person who decides at the table after three drinks is operating from a compromised one.

Pre-decide. Pre-commit. Pre-load. Pre-exit. Those four words apply to restaurants, holidays, travel, social events, and grocery shopping alike. Decide when you're clear—not when you're compromised.

Rule 4—Below 30 Grams of Carbs for Two to Three Days, and the Hunger Collapses.

Not gradually. Dramatically. When carbohydrate intake drops below 30 grams a day, most adults shift from glucose dependence to fat burning within forty-eight to seventy-two hours. Insulin drops to baseline, and the constant hunger signal that was firing every ninety minutes goes quiet.

After that point, you're no longer fighting hunger—you're only retraining habits, and habits respond to environment design. Three hard days. Then the whole project gets dramatically easier.

Rule 5—Starches Are Sugar. Read Total Carbs, Not the Sugar Line.

Bread, pasta, rice, potatoes—these often produce a higher blood sugar response than table sugar. A label that says "zero sugar" but shows 30 grams of total carbohydrate is showing you 30 grams of sugar wearing a different name.

Ignore the front of the package and the "natural," "wholesome," "heart-healthy" marketing. Flip it over. Total carbohydrate, minus fiber, equals net carbs—and net carbs are the number that matters. Over 5 grams per realistic serving, and the food is working against you.

Rule 6—Real Meat Satisfies. Engineered Food Does Not.

A six-ounce steak with butter satisfies hunger for four to six hours. A protein bar with the same protein content satisfies for sixty to ninety minutes—and then triggers more hunger than it relieved, because the sweeteners and binders spike insulin and restart the craving cycle.

Real meat isn't just a protein source. It's a satiety system. The protein bar is processed food wearing a health costume. Choose real food. Always.

Rule 7—Fat Is the Off Switch. Add More Than Feels Normal.

Cutting carbohydrates without adding fat is the most common reason low-carb attempts fail inside a week. The body is hunting for its satiety signal; if glucose isn't providing it, fat has to. When the fat isn't there, the hunger continues—and the person decides low-carb "doesn't work for them." It works. They just didn't add enough fat.

Butter on the vegetables. Fatty cuts over lean. Olive oil over everything. Avocado at every opportunity. Full-fat dairy. Eggs cooked in butter, not spray. Add fat until the meal satisfies completely—then you've found the right amount.

Rule 8—The Morning Sets Everything Downstream.

What happens in the first sixty minutes after waking sets the hormonal and neurological baseline for the rest of the day. Morning light within thirty minutes anchors the circadian clock. No phone in the first hour protects the cognitive baseline. Protein instead of carbohydrate at breakfast eliminates the

3:00 p.m. crash before it starts. A short walk deploys movement before the sedentary environment takes over.

Fix the morning and the rest of the day is easier. Lose it to the phone, the cereal, and the indoor light, and you spend the day trying to recover from the deficit.

Rule 9—Duration Beats Intensity as the Primary Stressor.

This applies to toxic exposure, EMF, screen time, sitting, cognitive load, and poor food alike. One big exposure event is rarely the problem. Continuous, low-grade, daily exposure—compounding over months and years—is what produces chronic disease.

So the goal isn't to avoid one bad day. It's to redesign the default, so the daily baseline is different. Architecture over heroics. Every time.

Rule 10—Exit Routes Matter as Much as Inputs.

Your body clears toxins, stress hormones, inflammatory compounds, and metabolic waste through five exit routes:

- Bile and bowel elimination
- Kidneys and hydration
- Skin and sweat
- Lungs and deep breathing
- Lymphatic movement

When these routes are open, the body handles a real load without crisis. When they're blocked—by constipation, dehydration, a sedentary day, shallow breathing, nutrient deficiency—load accumulates no matter how clean the inputs are. Support the exits with the same intention you give the inputs: move, hydrate, sweat occasionally, breathe deeply, and eat the glycine-rich foods that keep the liver pathways running.

Rule 11—The Biological Minimum. When Everything Else Fails, Protect These Five.

On the worst travel day, the most chaotic holiday, the most stressful week—when every other protocol has collapsed—protect only these:

- Morning sunlight within thirty to sixty minutes of waking
- At least one meal built around protein
- Phone out of the bedroom at night
- A walk at some point during the day
- Water with electrolytes

These five maintain enough biological stability to prevent the multi-day spiral that turns one hard day into three hard weeks. They require almost no willpower, they work in any environment, and they keep the platform stable enough that recovery is one good day away instead of one month away.

Rule 12—Reset Immediately. Not Monday. Now.

The most dangerous moment in any health protocol is not the indulgence. It's the decision that comes after it. One meal never causes collapse. One holiday never destroys months of progress. What destroys progress is the decision to extend the deviation—"I already blew it, so I might as well keep going until Monday."

The reset rule is simple: Whatever happened last night, this morning is a new morning. Sunlight. Walk. Protein. Water. Immediately. No punishment, no aggressive compensation, no skipping meals to make up for it. Return to baseline immediately—every time, without drama.

The Reference Protocols

Pull these out when you need them. They're situation-specific operating systems, not rules to memorize.

A note on how these protocols line up with the nine environments: they don't—at least not one to one, and that's deliberate. The nine environments are the diagnosis; they tell you which part of your life is feeding your biology the wrong signal. The protocols here are the prescription—situation-by-situation moves for actually changing those signals. One protocol often serves several environments at once: The Food Environment Reset steadies your microbiome and your nutrients along with your food, and the Sleep & Light protocol does as much for your cognitive environment as for your sleep. A single environment, in turn, may draw on several protocols. So don't go looking for one protocol per chapter. Find the environment that scored highest in your audit, start with its Start Here move, and pull in whichever protocols serve it.

Protocol 1—The Food Environment Reset

Use this when starting from scratch, or after a period of drift.

The One Question That Determines Where You Start

On a scale of 1 to 10, how willing are you to make changes if those changes create a massive effect on your health? Not how willing you are to read about it—how willing you are to actually do it.

If you answered 8–10—The Purge. Remove everything that works against you in one organized week. Get below 30 grams of carbohydrate a day and let the biology switch. Three to four hard days, then the hunger collapses and everything after is habit work, not biological battle.

If you answered 5–7—The Gradient. One phase at a time, two weeks per phase. Sugary drinks out first. Clear the counter second. Switch breakfast third. Work through the meals until you arrive at the same destination—more slowly, with less initial discomfort.

If you answered 1–4—The Foundation. Don't change your food yet. Do these for two weeks, then re-score (you'll likely be at a 6 or 7), then move to the Gradient:

- Walk 15 minutes after dinner every day
- Get morning sunlight within thirty minutes of waking
- Stop eating after 7:00 p.m.
- Replace all sugary drinks with water
- Eat eggs cooked in butter for breakfast

The Purge—What Leaves, What Comes In

Everything that leaves: all forms of sugar in every disguise (see the list below); all refined starches—bread, pasta, rice, potatoes, cereal, crackers, chips, tortillas, flour; seed oils—canola, soybean, corn, sunflower, safflower, vegetable; packaged foods with more than five ingredients; liquid calories—juice, soda, sports drinks, sweetened anything.

Everything that comes in: real animal protein at every meal—beef, chicken thighs, pork, lamb, fatty fish, eggs, organ meat; real fat—butter, olive oil, avocado oil, animal fats, avocados, olives, full-fat cheese, heavy cream, nuts in moderation; above-ground vegetables—leafy greens, cruciferous, asparagus, zucchini, peppers, mushrooms, fermented vegetables; pantry anchors—sea salt, apple cider vinegar, real mustard, avocado-oil mayo, bone broth, coconut aminos, unsweetened sparkling water.

The 60+ Disguise Names of Sugar

- **The –ose family:** sucrose, dextrose, fructose, glucose, maltose, galactose, lactose.
- **The syrups:** corn syrup, high-fructose corn syrup, brown rice syrup, malt syrup, agave, cane syrup, oat syrup, golden syrup.
- **The "healthy-sounding" ones:** coconut sugar, date sugar, palm sugar, turbinado, demerara, muscovado, organic cane sugar, evaporated cane juice, fruit juice concentrate, panela, jaggery.
- **The industrial ones (most dangerous—they hide in**

"sugar-free" products): maltodextrin, dextrin, modified corn starch, modified food starch, polydextrose, isomaltose, crystalline fructose, oligofructose.

Maltodextrin has a higher glycemic index than table sugar. A product labeled "sugar-free" can be loaded with it.

How to Read a Label in 15 Seconds

- Ignore the front entirely. Flip it over.
- Total carbohydrate, minus fiber, equals net carbs.
- Net carbs over 5 grams per realistic serving—put it back.
- More than 5 ingredients, any sugar-disguise name, or any seed oil—put it back.

The Satiety Hierarchy

Food	**How long it holds you**
Fatty meat—ribeye, chicken thighs, salmon	4 to 6 hours
Eggs cooked in butter	4 to 5 hours
Full-fat cheese and dairy	3 to 4 hours
Avocado, olives, nuts	about 3 hours
Lean protein alone	about 2 hours
Vegetables alone	about 1 hour
Starch and grain	60 to 90 min—then craving more
Sugar and refined carbs	30 to 60 min—then ravenous
Protein bars	60 to 90 min—then more cravings than before

The Substitute Map

Keep the rituals your family expects, without the biological cost.

Instead of	Reach for
Pizza	Cauliflower-crust or fathead-dough pizza
Pasta	Zucchini noodles, shirataki, hearts-of-palm pasta
Rice	Cauliflower rice, shirataki rice
Bread	Almond-flour bread, cloud bread, 90-second bread
Mashed potatoes	Mashed cauliflower with butter and cream
Chips	Cheese crisps, pork rinds, Parmesan crisps
Ice cream	Heavy cream + erythritol + vanilla, churned frozen
Cookies	Almond-flour cookies, fat bombs
Pancakes	Almond-flour or cream-cheese pancakes
Soda	Sparkling water with stevia and natural flavoring

Find recipes at drberg.com—search by food name. Print the top thirty and keep them in a binder in the kitchen.

The Two Tactics That Work Even on Your Worst Day

Eat in the right order. At any meal, whatever's on the plate: protein first, vegetables second, fat alongside, carbs last if present. This one sequencing change cuts the post-meal blood sugar spike by 30 to 50 percent, even with the same total food.

Walk after the meal. Ten to fifteen minutes. Muscles pull glucose out of the bloodstream without insulin, cutting the spike another 30 to 40 percent on top of the sequencing. Combined, these two tactics roughly halve the metabolic damage of a high-carb meal. Use them on the wedding day, the holiday meal, the family dinner you can't control.

The Predictable Vulnerability Windows

Window	What's happening, and the defense
3:00 to 4:00 p.m.	A high-carb lunch crashed your blood sugar. Defense: a protein-and-fat lunch with no refined carbs eliminates the crash before it starts.
Post-dinner, pre-bed	Cortisol drops, willpower depletes, dopamine seeks a final hit. Defense: kitchen closed—lights off at a set time, counters cleared, teeth brushed as the final friction.
After alcohol	Blood sugar drops while inhibitions drop. Defense: protein and fat before any drinks, one to two maximum, no sugar in the house when drinking happens.
After poor sleep	Reward sensitivity to sugar rises 30 to 50 percent after one short night. Defense: pre-decide it's a high-vulnerability day—extra fat at breakfast, walk earlier, bed earlier.
Emotional stress	Cortisol spikes, then crashes. Defense: walk first, before deciding anything about food. The walk is the regulation the food was trying to provide.

Protocol 2—The Grocery Store

The most upstream intervention in your food environment. What doesn't enter the house can't be eaten in the house.

Before You Go

- Never enter hungry—eat protein and fat thirty to sixty minutes before. Hunger in a grocery store is a decision-making impairment.

- Make the list at home, not in the store. The list is the decision; the store is just the execution.

The Navigation Rules

- Shop the perimeter first and almost exclusively—produce, meat, eggs, dairy. The interior aisles are where the engineered food lives.
- Go to interior aisles only for targeted items—olive oil, vinegar, canned fish, spices, sparkling water. Go directly, grab it, leave. Don't browse.
- Spend more time in the meat section than anywhere else. Fatty cuts over lean—chicken thighs over breast, 80/20 ground beef over 90/10, salmon, sardines, mackerel. Ask what came in fresh. Buy for the week.

At Every Label—The 15-Second Rule

- Flip it. Total carbs minus fiber. Over 5 grams net per realistic serving—back it goes.
- More than five ingredients, any seed oil, any sugar-disguise name—back it goes.

The Defensive Stocking List

Keep these in the house permanently, so when hunger hits there's always a compliant option in reach:

- Hard-boiled eggs already made, full-fat cheese, olives, sardines in olive oil

- Nuts—macadamia and pecans first, almonds third—and avocados every trip
- Butter always, sauerkraut in the fridge, sparkling water stocked

Protocol 3—The Restaurant

The mistake is deciding at the table. Every decision gets made before you walk in.

Before You Arrive

- Look at the menu online first. Pre-commit to three things: the protein, the vegetable, the drink. Arrive having already ordered in your head.
- Classify the event in advance—structured (stay aligned), flexible (one pre-decided indulgence), or intentional indulgence (rare, planned, no guilt, no extension). Never decide the category after you've sat down.
- If you're unsure about the food quality, eat a small protein snack before leaving. Arriving hungry is a loss of control before you're through the door.

At the Table

- Order water immediately—hydration reduces impulsive ordering.
- Decide in advance whether this is a bread-basket occasion. Don't "just have one" as an unconsidered grab.
- Build the meal around protein—steak, fish, chicken,

lamb, eggs—never base it on carbs and add protein as an afterthought.

- Request modifications calmly and without explanation: "without the sauce," "cooked in butter if possible," "no fries—double vegetables." No lecture owed.
- Restaurant portions are large—split the plate in half mentally before you start. Eat slowly, pause at the half-way point. You can always eat more; you rarely need to.

Alcohol

- Decide the limit before the first drink—none, one, or two maximum.
- Never drink before food. Protein first, then alcohol. One glass of water between each drink.
- Never stack alcohol and dessert in the same evening—choose one indulgence axis.

After

- Walk ten to fifteen minutes—not optional if a carbohydrate was consumed.
- No late-night screen drift afterward; it compounds the metabolic damage straight into the sleep window.

Protocol 4—Holidays

You don't "stay disciplined" during holidays. You pre-decide, pre-load, pre-commit, and pre-exit.

Before the Event

- Eat protein, fat, and fiber before leaving. Never arrive hungry.
- Walk or move lightly before the event—it improves insulin sensitivity and lowers craving intensity at the table.
- Classify the event in advance: controlled, flexible (one pre-decided deviation), or rare intentional indulgence (full departure, no extension, immediate reset the next morning).

At the Table

- First plate: half protein, half vegetables. Then sit.
- Pause ten to fifteen minutes before any second plate or dessert.
- Don't hover at the food table—plate your food, sit with people, eat it, and stop. Holiday tables are continuous-eating environments by design.
- If dessert happens, it happens last, one portion, no stacking with alcohol.

When Pushed

- "It looks great—I'm just pacing myself." Short, calm, closed. No nutrition lecture, no debate.
- "I'm good for now," for alcohol pressure—repeat without elaboration.
- "I feel better this way," for any comment about your choices. Smile, move on.

The 3-Night Rule

- Never allow three consecutive destabilized nights. One late night with alcohol and poor sleep—the next night must be clean. One event never causes collapse; three in a row produce the drift that takes a month to undo.

The Next Morning

- Morning sunlight immediately. Walk. High-protein breakfast. No punishment fasting, no shame.
- Return to baseline immediately—not Monday, not after the holidays. The morning after the event is a new morning.

Protocol 5—Travel

You can't control everything. You control five things—light, movement, protein, sleep window, and alcohol stacking—and those prevent 80 percent of the damage.

Before You Leave

- Lock your wake time three to five days before travel, especially across time zones. The wake time is the anchor—not the bedtime.
- Reduce stimulation forty-eight hours before: no late nights, no heavy alcohol, no high-intensity training.
- Pack protein snacks—jerky, nuts, protein packets—and electrolytes. Never rely on airport food.

Airport and Flight

- Never arrive hungry. Walk the terminal ten to twenty minutes—it prevents the blood sugar instability and circulation stagnation of sitting at the gate.
- Avoid airport alcohol by default. Hydrate aggressively in the air—water every hour, electrolytes added, no sugary drinks.
- Move every hour on the flight: stand, stretch, walk the aisle.
- Match destination time immediately. Daytime when you land—stay awake. Nighttime—attempt sleep on the plane. Don't live in the in-between time.

Arrival

- Sunlight within one hour of landing—outside, even for ten minutes. This resets the clock faster than anything else.
- Walk after arrival. Protein as the first meal at the destination.
- No long nap—twenty to thirty minutes maximum if exhausted, then push through to local bedtime.

Hotel Environment

- On entering: close the blackout curtains, lower the thermostat, move the phone off the bedside, unplug glowing alarm clocks. Redesign the room before relaxing.
- Close the minibar. Don't browse it.

Food & Return Home

- Anchor one protein-and-vegetable meal per day, non-negotiable, regardless of the other meals.
- Avoid continuous grazing from airport snacks, lobby food, and conference trays. Use tourism as movement, not transportation.
- First twenty-four hours home: full reset—morning sunlight, long walk, clean meals, early bedtime. No "recovery junk," no extending the travel behavior into day one back.

Protocol 6—Stress Eating

Stress eating is a regulation strategy. Remove the food without replacing the regulation, and it comes back stronger.

Identify the Type

- **Acute emotional spike**—a sudden argument or overwhelm. The urge is fast and intense.
- **Chronic cortisol fatigue**—a long workday, decision fatigue, sleep deprivation. The urge is slow-building and persistent.
- **Dopamine boredom**—late night, scrolling, idle time, TV. The urge is stimulation-driven, not hunger-driven.

The 90-Second Interrupt

- Stand up immediately and leave the room. Change your posture and location—stress eating thrives in stillness.
- Take ten slow breaths: four seconds in, six seconds out.

- Set a ten-minute timer. Most urges fade within ten minutes once you've inserted friction and movement. If you still want food after, decide intentionally—not reactively.

The Replacement

- **For acute stress:** physical discharge—a five-minute brisk walk, cold water on the face, push-ups, brief outdoor exposure.
- **For chronic fatigue:** protein if genuinely hungry, electrolytes and water, a twenty-minute nap, a short walk.
- **For dopamine boredom:** replace stimulation with action—clean something, call someone, go outside, read a physical book.

If You Eat Anyway, and Prevention

- It's one event, not a collapse. Plate it, sit, eat slowly and intentionally—never standing, from a bag, or in front of the open fridge. After any sugar or carb, anchor the next meal in protein.
- Prevention is removal: no candy bowl on the desk, no visible chips, no open snack basket. A food you can't see requires a conscious decision; a food you can see triggers eating without one.
- The after-work transition is the highest-risk window. Interrupt the cortisol carryover before it reaches the kitchen—a walk before entering the house, five minutes of breathing in the car, changing clothes the moment you arrive.

Protocol 7—The Workspace

The workspace is an environment. Design it the same way you designed your food environment.

The Non-Negotiables

- Movement alarm every forty-five to sixty minutes—stand and move through space for five minutes. Not stretching at the desk. Moving. Set the alarm; don't rely on memory.
- At the break, undo the desk shape—a half-kneeling hip-flexor lunge, a chest opener, a chin tuck. Two or three minutes reverses the compressions sitting builds in.
- Screen top at or below eye level. On a laptop at a desk, get a stand and a separate keyboard—wrong height is a structural injury in slow motion.
- Deep work blocks capped at ninety minutes, then a real break—outside if possible, no screens, actual movement.
- Phone in another room during deep work. Not face down on the desk—in another room. Its mere presence measurably reduces available cognitive capacity, even off.

The Vision Reset

- Every sixty minutes: look as far away as possible—window, hallway, outside—then back to something close. Alternate five to ten times, sixty seconds. The single best thing for ciliary-muscle flexibility. Do it every time the movement alarm goes off.
- Every few minutes at a screen: one slow, full, deliberate

blink—not a flutter. It re-wets the tear film screen work evaporates.

The EMF Minimums

- Never put a laptop on your lap.
- Phone off the body during sustained work—on the desk, not in the pocket.
- Distance from routers and power bricks—two extra feet produces a dramatic drop in field intensity.
- Phone charges in another room at night, every night.

The Cognitive Decompression Rule

When a sustained session ends, move before any other screen. Walk first—give the cortisol that built during the session a physical outlet before introducing more input. This is the difference between ending the day recovered and ending it wired.

Protocol 8—The Sleep and Light Environment

Light is instruction. Your body uses it to know what time it is—when to activate, when to repair, when to shut down.

The Morning Sequence—Non-Negotiable

- Outdoor light within thirty to sixty minutes of waking. No sunglasses for the first exposure. Minimum ten minutes; twenty to forty-five is better. Before coffee, before the phone, before anything digital.
- Same wake time every day—thirty minutes of variance maximum, weekends included. Two hours of weekend

drift produces Monday jet lag every week for life. The clock stabilizes from the wake time, not the bedtime.

The Evening Sequence

- Overhead lights off at or near sunset—lamps only, warm spectrum. Overhead LED at night is one of the primary circadian disruptors in the modern home. Pre-set dimmers or lamp timers so it happens without a decision.
- Screens end two to three hours before sleep, ideally. Night mode is not a solution—it lowers blue frequency but not brightness, and melanopsin responds to brightness too. It's not the same as putting the screen away.

The Bedroom—Zero Compromise

- Not dim. Dark. Blackout curtains, every LED covered or removed—TV standby light, power-strip indicator, charging light. The retina detects light even through closed eyelids.
- Phone out of the bedroom. Analog alarm clock; phone charges in another room. Reaching for it during a night waking triggers alertness, light, and cortisol.
- Room temperature 65 to 68°F. Core temperature has to drop to initiate and maintain deep sleep; a warm room fights the shutdown signal.

The Food–Sleep Connection

- Kitchen closed three to four hours before bed. A late meal raises blood sugar, then drops it around 2:00 to

4:00 a.m., triggering an adrenaline release that wakes you for "no reason." The late meal is the reason. The 3:00 a.m. wakeups resolve for most people within one to two weeks of eating earlier.

The Fourteen-Day Clock Reset

When sleep is significantly disrupted, enforce only these five for fourteen days. No supplements, no other changes. Most people see dramatic improvement in seven to ten days:

- Fixed wake time every day
- Morning outdoor light within thirty minutes
- Phone out of the bedroom
- Kitchen closed three to four hours before bed
- Overhead lights off after sunset

The Master Chart

One page. The governing logic of the whole book.

Environment	The primary problem	The primary fix
Food	Distorted signals—industrial food overrides biology	Real food, fill the gaps, redesign what's visible
Light & Sleep	Dim days and bright nights erase the clock	Morning outdoor light, dark bedroom
Movement	Sedentary work undone by one gym session	Move every 45 minutes, walk after meals
Chemical	Continuous low-level load exceeds clearance	Reduce inputs, support the exit routes
Microbiome	Ecological collapse from antibiotics and sterility	Fermented food daily, fiber diversity

Environment	The primary problem	The primary fix
Cognitive	Dopamine hijack by engineered stimulation	Delete, don't moderate; protect the quiet
Social	Stimulation without regulation	Depth over breadth; real presence
Workspace	Eight hours inverting every biological signal	45-minute rule, vision resets, light
Nutrients	Missing machinery despite adequate calories	Organ meat, eggs, fatty fish, magnesium

The universal rule across all nine:

Fix the architecture. The behavior follows.

PART III
RESOURCES

The wellnessMAP App

Everything in this book is a system you have to run—and running it is far easier with the right tool. That is why we built the wellnessMAP app.

It takes what you have read here and turns it into something you can actually do. Your audit, your Start Here moves, the protocols in Part II—all of it becomes simple, trackable steps instead of a stack of notes and good intentions.

It also learns what works for you specifically. As you make changes and log how you respond, it gets better at telling you which moves are actually moving your numbers—because no two people respond to the same environment in exactly the same way.

And here is the part I am most excited about: You are not doing this alone. Combined across everyone using it, your experience helps surface patterns none of us could see by ourselves—which changes tend to help which kinds of people, and in what order. You benefit from everyone who came before you, and the next person benefits from you. That is the real power of doing this together instead of alone.

You can find wellnessMAP at **wellnessmap.ai**.

And you can take the Health Lever Quiz—the online version of the Environment Audit from the start of this book—at **drberg.com/health-lever-quiz**.

The *L. reuteri* Yogurt Recipe

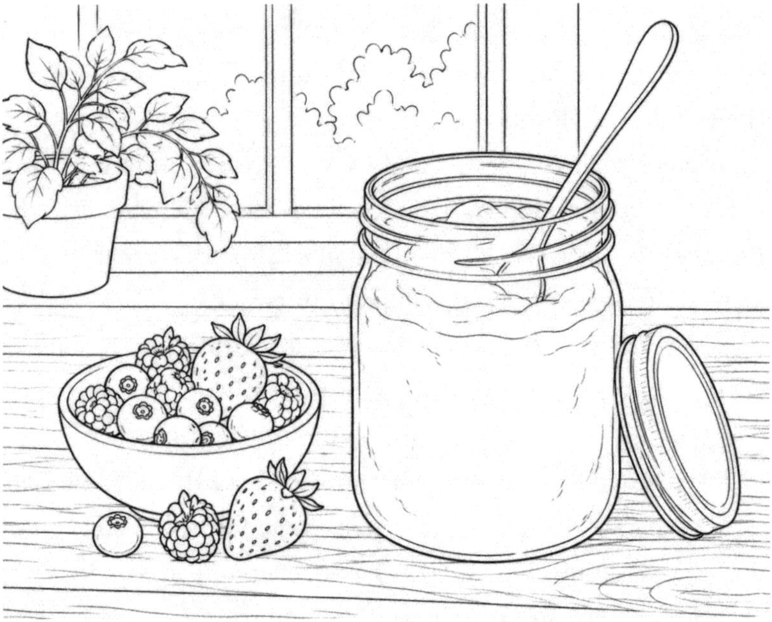

Back in Chapter 7, I mentioned the *L. reuteri* yogurt I learned about from Dr. William Davis. Here's how I make it. It's adapted from his protocol—his book *Super Gut* has the full background—but this is enough to get you started.

What makes it different from regular yogurt is two things. First, the culture: Most yogurt doesn't contain *L. reuteri* at all, so you have to seed it yourself, and the easiest source is BioGaia

Gastrus tablets, which carry two well-studied *L. reuteri* strains. Second, the ferment is long. Where ordinary yogurt sets in about eight hours, this one ferments for thirty-six hours at a gentle temperature, to let the *L. reuteri* multiply into the huge numbers that make it worth eating. You also feed it a prebiotic fiber so the bacteria have something to grow on.

You'll need:

- 1 quart (about 1 liter) of half-and-half—the higher fat makes it thick and gives the bacteria what they like; whole milk works but sets thinner.
- 10 BioGaia Gastrus tablets, crushed to a powder—for your first batch only. After that, you save 2 tablespoons of finished yogurt as the starter for the next one.
- 2 tablespoons of inulin or another prebiotic fiber—this is the food that lets the culture reach high counts.
- A yogurt maker or sous vide setup that holds a steady 100°F (about 37 to 40°C). This matters: most off-the-shelf yogurt makers run too hot—110°F and up—and will kill the culture over thirty-six hours. Steady, gentle temperature is the one piece of equipment worth getting right. My favorite yogurt maker is the Ultimate Yogurt Maker. You can find it here: www.amazon.com/ultimate.

Method:

1. Whisk the inulin into a few tablespoons of the half-and-half until smooth and lump-free, then stir it back into the rest.

2. For the first batch, stir in the crushed tablets. For every batch after, stir in 2 tablespoons of yogurt saved from the last one.
3. Pour into clean jars and ferment at 100°F for 36 hours. Don't rush it—the long, slow ferment is the whole point.
4. It should come out thick and tangy, sometimes with a little separation, which is normal. Chill it, and save 2 tablespoons in a clean jar in your refrigerator as the starter for your next batch.

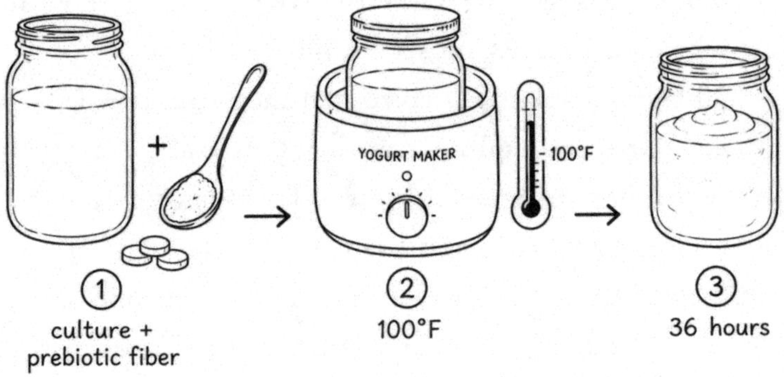

How to eat it: Start small—a couple of tablespoons a day—and build up as your gut adjusts. Some people notice the effects on mood, sleep, and sociability I described in Chapter 7; some feel less. Either way, you're delivering a keystone microbe most of us lost a long time ago.

One note: This is food, not medicine. If you're immune-compromised or dealing with a serious gut condition, run it by your doctor first. And if a batch ever smells off, looks moldy, or turns colors, throw it out and start fresh. Trust your nose.

Where to source *L. reuteri*:

https://www.biogaia.com/products/osfortis

https://www.oxiceutics.com/products/myreuteri

Glossary of Terms

Plain-English definitions for every scientific and technical term used in the book.

When you hit a word you don't recognize, this is where you find it.

A note on this glossary

This book is written to be understood without a medical degree. But it does use specific scientific terms—because precision matters, and vague language leads to vague results. Every term listed here appears in the book. Definitions are intentionally plain and short. The goal is clarity, not a medical encyclopedia.

— A —

Adrenaline (Epinephrine)

A stress hormone released by the adrenal glands in response to danger, low blood sugar, or intense emotion. It raises heart rate, raises blood glucose, and prepares the body for physical action. In the modern stress cycle, adrenaline gets released—but the physical action never comes.

→ *See Chapter 3—the incomplete stress cycle.*

Ancestral Mismatch

The gap between the environment your body was designed for—through 2.5 million years of evolution—and the modern environment it is actually living in. When those two environments are far apart, your biology gets false signals. Most of the chronic health problems described in this book are expressions of that mismatch.

→ *The central thesis of this book. See Before We Begin.*

Autophagy

The body's built-in cellular recycling process. During fasting or low-calorie periods, cells break down and repurpose their own damaged or worn-out components—organelles, misfolded proteins, old cellular debris—and use them for fuel or rebuilding. Literally means "self-eating" in Greek. This is one of the main reasons fasting is biologically useful: it turns on the cleanup system.

→ *See Chapter 1—The Fasting Absence Principle.*

—B—

Beta-Carotene

A plant pigment found in orange and yellow vegetables—carrots, sweet potatoes, squash. The body can convert it into vitamin A, but conversion is slow and highly variable. Not the same as preformed retinol (the form found in animal foods). Beta-carotene does not carry the same risks as high-dose preformed vitamin A.

→ *See Chapter 1—organ meats and nutrient density.*

Bliss Point

A food-science term for the precise combination of sugar, fat, salt, and texture that maximizes how much pleasure a food produces—and minimizes the signal to stop eating. Food manufacturers use research and development specifically to find and engineer this point. It is not accidental. It is optimized.

→ *See Chapter 1—engineered food.*

Blood Glucose (Blood Sugar)

The amount of glucose—a simple sugar—circulating in your bloodstream at any moment. The body tightly regulates this level. When it rises too high (after a large meal or sugary drink), insulin is released to bring it down. When it drops too low (after a long gap without eating, or in the night), adrenaline is released to push it back up. Chronically elevated blood glucose is the foundation of metabolic disease.

→ *Referenced throughout Chapters 1 and 2.*

Blue Light

Short-wavelength light in the 400–490 nanometer range. The morning sky is naturally rich in blue light, and the cells in the retina that set your circadian clock are most sensitive to it. Modern LED lighting and screens emit significant blue light—which at night sends a false "it is midday" signal to your brain, suppressing melatonin and disrupting sleep.

→ *See Chapter 2—the 480nm problem.*

— C —

Cephalic Phase of Digestion

The first phase of digestion—the one that starts before food even reaches the stomach. It is triggered by chewing, tasting, smelling, and even seeing food. It primes saliva production, stomach acid, and early satiety hormones. Soft, pre-blended food reduces this phase significantly, meaning the brain gets less of a "food is coming" warning signal—and tends to register fullness later.

→ *See Chapter 1—texture and chewing.*

Circadian Clock (Circadian Rhythm)

The internal twenty-four-hour biological timer that governs virtually every system in the body—hormones, metabolism, immune function, digestion, body temperature, and sleep. Every cell runs its own version of this clock. The master clock sits in the brain (the SCN) and keeps all the cellular clocks synchronized using light as its primary input signal.

→ *See Chapter 2—the full timing system.*

Cofactor

A helper molecule—often a mineral or vitamin—that an enzyme needs in order to do its job. Without the cofactor, the enzyme is structurally present but functionally inactive. For example, magnesium is a cofactor for the enzymes that activate vitamin D. Zinc is a cofactor for the vitamin D receptor. If the cofactor is missing, the process it enables does not happen.

→ *See Chapter 9—nutrients as infrastructure.*

Collagen

The most abundant protein in the human body. It forms the structural scaffolding of skin, tendons, ligaments, cartilage, bone, and the gut lining. Produced by the body using glycine (from connective tissue and bone broth) and vitamin C. Modern diets, which focus on muscle meat and skip connective tissue cuts, are often low in the building blocks collagen requires.

→ *See Chapter 1—what is missing from the modern food supply.*

Copper

A trace mineral essential for iron metabolism, collagen formation, immune function, and antioxidant defense. Abundant in organ meats—particularly beef liver. Deficient in most modern diets, which rely on muscle meat alone.

→ *See Chapter 1—nutrient density and organ meats.*

Cortisol

The body's primary stress hormone, produced by the adrenal glands. In the morning, it rises sharply to wake you up and give you energy—this is normal and healthy. Through the day it should taper gradually. At night, it should be low, allowing sleep and repair. When the light environment is disrupted, or stress is chronic, cortisol stays elevated into the evening—blocking deep sleep and keeping fat storage high.

→ *See Chapters 2 and 3.*

Cortisol Awakening Response (CAR)
The sharp spike in cortisol that occurs in the first twenty to thirty minutes after waking. It is amplified by morning bright light. This pulse sets the metabolic and immune tone for the entire day. When the light environment is poor—no bright morning light—the CAR is blunted, leading to flat energy, immune suppression, and disrupted metabolism all day.
→ *See Chapter 2.*

— D —

Deep Sleep (Slow-Wave Sleep)
The most physically restorative stage of sleep. During slow-wave sleep, the brain produces slow, synchronized electrical activity, growth hormone is released in its largest pulse of the day, and the body does its primary tissue repair—muscle, bone, collagen, immune cells. Disrupted by high evening cortisol, poor sleep timing, and late-night eating.
→ *See Chapter 2.*

Dopamine
A neurotransmitter involved in motivation, reward, focus, and the drive to pursue goals. It is released in anticipation of reward, not just during reward—which is why phone notifications, social media, and engineered food are so compelling. Chronically overstimulated dopamine systems lose sensitivity over time, requiring more stimulation to feel the same effect.
→ *See Chapter 6—the cognitive-dopamine environment.*

—E—

Endocrine Disruptor

A chemical—natural or synthetic—that interferes with the body's hormonal signaling system. Endocrine disruptors can mimic hormones, block hormone receptors, or alter the rate at which hormones are produced or broken down. Common sources: PFAS-coated cookware, plastics, synthetic fragrance, pesticides, and personal care products.

→ *See Chapter 4—the chemical environment.*

Enzyme

A protein that speeds up a specific chemical reaction in the body. Enzymes are the workers of biology—they convert one substance into another, break things down, or build things up. Most require cofactors (minerals or vitamins) to function. Without the right cofactor, the enzyme is present but inactive.

—F—

Fat-Burning Pathways

The metabolic processes by which the body breaks down stored fat (triglycerides) and uses it for energy. These pathways are activated when insulin is low—during fasting, sleep, or low-carbohydrate eating. When insulin is chronically elevated (from frequent eating, sugar, processed food), fat-burning is suppressed regardless of calorie intake.

→ *See Chapter 1.*

Fight-or-Flight Response

The body's emergency activation system, governed by the sympathetic nervous system. In response to a perceived threat, adrenaline and cortisol flood the body: heart rate rises, blood glucose spikes, muscles tense, digestion pauses, and the body prepares for intense physical action. In modern life, this response is triggered by emails, traffic, and deadlines—but the physical discharge that should follow never happens.

→ *See Chapter 3.*

Forward Head Posture

A postural pattern in which the head sits forward of the shoulder line—typically caused by looking down at screens or hunching toward a monitor. For every inch the head moves forward, the effective weight it places on the cervical spine increases by approximately ten pounds. A head at two to four inches forward posture adds twenty to thirty pounds of load to the neck and upper back.

→ *See Chapter 8—workspace environment.*

— G —

Ghrelin

Often called the "hunger hormone." Produced primarily in the stomach, ghrelin signals the brain that it is time to eat—it rises before meals and drops after eating. Sleep deprivation significantly raises ghrelin, which is one reason poor sleep drives food cravings the next day.

→ *See Chapter 2—the sleep-food connection.*

Glucose

The simplest form of sugar, and the body's primary fast-burning fuel. Derived from carbohydrates in food. Circulates in the bloodstream as blood glucose. Regulated by insulin (which moves it into cells) and glucagon and adrenaline (which raise it when it drops too low).

Glycine

An amino acid—a building block of protein—that is abundant in connective tissue, bone broth, and organ meats, but almost absent from muscle meat alone. Glycine is essential for collagen production, liver detoxification, and regulation of the nervous system. A diet based on muscle meat only is almost always glycine-deficient.

→ *See Chapter 1—what is missing from the modern food supply.*

Growth Hormone

A hormone produced by the pituitary gland that drives tissue repair, muscle growth, bone maintenance, and fat metabolism. Its largest daily pulse is released in the first hours of deep slow-wave sleep. Disrupted sleep—especially from poor light environments or late eating—cuts this pulse short, impairing overnight repair.

→ *See Chapter 2.*

—H—

Hedonic Response

The pleasure signal generated by eating—particularly engineered food. The term describes the brain's reward reaction to food inputs: how much it wants more, how well it overrides fullness signals, and how strongly the memory of the food drives future seeking behavior. Food scientists design for maximum hedonic response. See also: bliss point.

→ *See Chapter 1.*

Hormone

A chemical messenger produced in one part of the body and carried through the bloodstream to give instructions to cells elsewhere. Hormones govern metabolism, sleep, reproduction, growth, stress response, hunger, and mood. The endocrine system produces and regulates hormones. Many modern environmental chemicals interfere with this signaling.

—I—

Industrial Seed Oils

Oils extracted from seeds and grains using high-heat, chemical, and industrial processing: soybean oil, corn oil, canola oil, sunflower oil, safflower oil, cottonseed oil. High in omega-6 fatty acids. The ratio of omega-6 to omega-3 in the ancestral diet was approximately 4:1. In the modern Western diet, this

ratio runs 15:1 to 20:1—primarily because seed oils are used in virtually all commercially prepared and restaurant food.
→ *See Chapter 1.*

Inflammation
The immune system's response to injury, infection, or perceived threat. Acute inflammation—a short burst in response to a specific injury—is healthy and necessary. Chronic low-grade inflammation—a persistent, low-level immune activation with no specific injury—underlies most modern chronic diseases, including heart disease, diabetes, autoimmune conditions, and neurodegeneration. Triggered by seed oils, high blood sugar, poor sleep, sedentary behavior, and chemical exposures.

Insulin
A hormone produced by the pancreas in response to rising blood glucose. Insulin's primary job is to move glucose from the bloodstream into cells for energy or storage. When insulin is high, fat burning is suppressed—the body stores rather than burns. Chronically elevated insulin (from frequent meals, sugar, processed food, and liquid calories) is the central driver of fat accumulation, metabolic syndrome, and type 2 diabetes.
→ *See Chapter 1—the insulin story.*

Insulin Sensitivity
How responsive your cells are to insulin's signal. High insulin sensitivity means cells respond quickly and efficiently—a small amount of insulin moves a lot of glucose. Low insulin sensitivity

(insulin resistance) means cells ignore the signal, requiring more and more insulin to do the same job. Movement, sleep, fasting, and real food all improve insulin sensitivity. Sitting, poor sleep, and processed food degrade it.
→ *See Chapters 1 and 3.*

Intermittent Fasting (IF)
An eating pattern in which food is consumed only within a defined time window each day, with the remaining hours spent fasting. Not a diet in the sense of restricting what you eat, but rather a pattern that restricts when. The fasting window allows insulin to fall, fat-burning pathways to activate, and autophagy to run. In this book, fasting is framed not as a strategy you impose, but as a natural result of a well-designed food environment.
→ *See Chapter 1—The Fasting Absence Principle.*

— K —

Ketosis
A metabolic state in which the body, running low on glucose, switches to burning fat as its primary fuel—producing ketone bodies as a byproduct. A natural, normal, and ancient metabolic state. Occurs during fasting, extended low-carbohydrate eating, or after a night of sleep. The human body is designed to move in and out of ketosis. The modern food environment, with its constant glucose supply, prevents this switch from ever happening.
→ *See Chapter 1—metabolic flexibility.*

Kinetic Chain

The interconnected system of joints, muscles, and connective tissue that work together to produce movement. In walking and running, the entire body participates—feet, ankles, knees, hips, core, shoulders, and arms all contribute. Sitting disrupts the kinetic chain by holding large portions of it in fixed, shortened positions for hours.

→ *See Chapter 3.*

—L—

Leptin

A hormone produced by fat cells that signals the brain that energy stores are sufficient—the "I have enough" signal. Sleep deprivation significantly lowers leptin, which, combined with the ghrelin increase, creates a powerful biological drive to overeat the following day. Poor sleep makes the food environment dramatically harder to manage.

→ *See Chapter 2.*

Lipoprotein Lipase (LPL)

An enzyme that sits on the walls of blood vessels and is critical for fat metabolism—it breaks down triglycerides in the blood so cells can use the fat for fuel. LPL activity drops dramatically within hours of continuous sitting, independently of whether you exercised earlier. This is the biochemical mechanism behind why "an hour at the gym cannot cancel eight hours of sitting."

→ *See Chapter 3.*

Lux

The unit used to measure how bright a light is as it falls on a surface. Ordinary indoor office lighting: 200–500 lux. A bright indoor environment: up to 1,000 lux. An overcast outdoor day: 10,000–20,000 lux. Direct midday sun: 50,000–130,000 lux. The circadian system requires bright light—well above indoor levels—to anchor properly.

→ *See Chapter 2.*

Lymphatic System

A network of vessels and nodes that moves lymph fluid—carrying immune cells, waste products, and cellular debris—through the body. Unlike blood, which has the heart as a pump, lymph has no pump of its own. It moves entirely through muscle contractions and body movement. A sedentary lifestyle means lymph stagnates—waste builds up, immune surveillance slows, and swelling can occur.

→ *See Chapter 3.*

— M —

Magnesium

A mineral involved in more than three hundred enzymatic reactions in the body, including those that activate vitamin D, produce ATP (cellular energy), regulate the nervous system, and maintain muscle function. An estimated 50 to 60 percent of Americans are below the recommended daily intake.

Deficiency signs include muscle cramps, restless sleep, tension, and wired-but-tired feelings at night.
→ *See Chapter 9.*

Melanopsin
A light-sensitive protein found in specialized cells in the retina (intrinsically photosensitive retinal ganglion cells). Melanopsin is most sensitive to blue light at around 480 nanometers—the wavelength dominant in morning sky light. When activated, it sends a signal to the SCN (master clock) that it is daytime, triggering the cascade of wakefulness hormones. Bright artificial light at night activates melanopsin inappropriately.
→ *See Chapter 2.*

Melatonin
A hormone produced by the pineal gland in response to darkness. It does not cause sleep—it signals that it is safe to sleep. Melatonin production is suppressed by light, particularly blue-wavelength light. Modern LED lighting at night can suppress melatonin by up to 50 percent. Taking a melatonin supplement without fixing the light environment is working against the biology, not with it.
→ *See Chapter 2.*

Metabolic Flexibility
The ability of the body to switch efficiently between burning glucose (sugar) and burning fat, depending on what fuel is available. A metabolically flexible person can go several

hours without eating without becoming shaky, foggy, or irritable—their body simply shifts to fat as fuel. A person eating frequently, with high insulin most of the day, loses this flexibility; they become dependent on frequent glucose top-ups.
→ *See Chapter 1—Question 5 of the audit.*

Metabolism
The sum total of all chemical reactions in the body that convert food and stored fuel into energy, and use that energy to run every biological process. Metabolism is not just a "fast" or "slow" setting—it is a complex, responsive system shaped significantly by when you eat, what you eat, how much you move, how you sleep, and what your light environment looks like.

Microbiome
The vast community of trillions of microorganisms—bacteria, fungi, viruses, and others—that live primarily in the large intestine. The gut microbiome is not a passive passenger; it produces neurotransmitters, trains the immune system, metabolizes certain nutrients, regulates inflammation, and influences mood and cognition. It is shaped by diet, medications, stress, sleep, and chemical exposures.
→ *See Chapter 5.*

Microbiome Diversity
The variety of different microbial species present in the gut. Higher diversity is consistently associated with better health outcomes—better immune function, lower inflammation,

more stable mood, and more resilient digestion. Diversity is primarily determined by dietary fiber variety: different fiber types feed different bacterial families.
→ *See Chapter 5.*

— N —

Nanometer (nm)
A unit of measurement equal to one billionth of a meter. Used to describe the wavelength of light. Visible light spans approximately 380–700nm. Blue light (the wavelength that sets the circadian clock) sits at approximately 480nm. Red and infrared light sit above 600nm. The wavelength determines how the body responds to a given light source.
→ *See Chapter 2.*

Neurotransmitter
A chemical messenger that carries signals between nerve cells (neurons) in the brain and nervous system. Major neurotransmitters mentioned in this book include dopamine (motivation, reward), serotonin (mood, well-being), and GABA (calm, inhibition). Many neurotransmitters are produced in or dependent on the gut microbiome.
→ *See Chapters 5 and 6.*

NSAIDs
Non-steroidal anti-inflammatory drugs. Common examples: ibuprofen (Advil, Motrin), naproxen (Aleve), aspirin. Widely

used for pain and inflammation. Regular or repeated use damages the gut lining, disrupts the intestinal barrier, and alters microbiome composition—contributing to leaky gut, microbiome dysbiosis, and systemic inflammation.
→ *See Chapter 5—medications and the microbiome.*

— O —

Omega-3 Fatty Acids
A family of polyunsaturated fats essential for cell membrane integrity, brain function, cardiovascular health, and anti-inflammatory signaling. The most biologically active forms (EPA and DHA) come from fatty fish, shellfish, and to some extent grass-fed animal products. The body cannot produce adequate amounts on its own—they must come from food or supplementation.
→ *See Chapter 9.*

Omega-6 Fatty Acids
A family of polyunsaturated fats found in abundance in industrial seed oils (soybean, corn, canola, sunflower). Pro-inflammatory in excess. The ancestral ratio of omega-6 to omega-3 was approximately 4:1. The modern Western ratio runs 15:1 to 20:1, primarily because seed oils are present in almost all commercially prepared food.
→ *See Chapter 1.*

Organ Meats

The internal organs of animals: liver, kidney, heart, brain, tongue, pancreas. Nutritionally far denser than muscle meat. Beef liver, in particular, is one of the highest-concentration sources of retinol (vitamin A), copper, zinc, B vitamins, and vitamin K2 available in any food. Removed from the default food supply as modern butchery moved to muscle-only cuts.

→ *See Chapter 1.*

—P—

Parabens

A family of synthetic preservatives used in personal care products, cosmetics, and some food products. Weak endocrine disruptors—they can mimic estrogen and interfere with hormonal signaling. Absorbed through the skin and detectable in blood and urine. Found in deodorant, lotion, shampoo, and makeup. Listed on labels as methylparaben, propylparaben, butylparaben, etc.

→ *See Chapter 4.*

PFAS (Per- and Polyfluoroalkyl Substances)

A family of thousands of synthetic chemicals used to make surfaces nonstick, water-resistant, and heat-resistant. Found in nonstick cookware (Teflon), food packaging, waterproof clothing, stain-resistant carpets, and firefighting foam. Called "forever chemicals" because they do not break down in the environment and accumulate in the human body over time.

Endocrine disruptors with documented links to thyroid disruption, immune suppression, hormonal imbalance, and certain cancers.
→ *See Chapter 4.*

Photopigment
A light-sensitive molecule found in cells of the retina. Different photopigments respond to different wavelengths of light. Rod cells use rhodopsin (for low-light, black-and-white vision). Cone cells use photopsins (for color vision). The specialized circadian-clock cells use melanopsin (for detecting blue light and setting the master clock).
→ *See Chapter 2.*

Phthalates
A group of synthetic chemicals used to make plastics soft and flexible, and to carry fragrance in personal care products and cleaning products. Found in soft plastic food packaging, vinyl flooring, fragranced lotions, shampoos, and air fresheners. Endocrine disruptors—they interfere with testosterone and estrogen signaling. Often listed on labels simply as "fragrance" or "parfum," because fragrance formulas are legally protected trade secrets.
→ *See Chapter 4.*

Probiotic
Live microorganisms—bacteria or yeasts—consumed in food or supplement form to support or replenish the gut microbiome.

Found naturally in fermented foods: yogurt, kefir, sauerkraut, kimchi, miso, tempeh. Probiotic supplements can help, but diversity of fermented food sources tends to deliver a wider variety of microbial strains.
→ *See Chapter 5.*

— R —

Receptor
A protein on or inside a cell that receives a specific chemical signal—like a lock that only one specific key can open. Hormones, neurotransmitters, and vitamins work by binding to their specific receptors, which then triggers a change in the cell's behavior. Some chemicals (including endocrine disruptors) can bind to receptors they were not designed for, sending false signals.

Retina
The light-sensitive layer at the back of the eye. Contains rod cells (low-light vision), cone cells (color vision), and a third type—intrinsically photosensitive retinal ganglion cells (ipRGCs)—that contain melanopsin and are responsible for sending light information to the master circadian clock in the brain. It is these cells, not the visual system, that set your biological time.
→ *See Chapter 2.*

Retinol (Preformed Vitamin A)

The biologically active, immediately usable form of vitamin A, found in animal foods—particularly liver, egg yolks, and full-fat dairy. Essential for vision, immune function, skin integrity, and gene expression. Distinct from beta-carotene, which is a plant-based precursor that the body must convert (inefficiently) into retinol. Largely absent from the modern food supply due to the shift away from organ meats.

→ *See Chapter 1.*

— S —

Satiety

The feeling of fullness and satisfaction after eating—the signal that enough food has been consumed. Satiety hormones include leptin (long-term energy status) and peptide YY and GLP-1 (short-term fullness signals triggered by eating). The cephalic phase of digestion begins the satiety process before food reaches the stomach. Liquid calories and soft foods bypass many of these signals.

→ *See Chapter 1.*

SCN (Suprachiasmatic Nucleus)

A tiny cluster of approximately twenty thousand neurons in the hypothalamus of the brain. The master circadian clock. Receives light signals from the retina (via melanopsin-containing cells), and uses them to synchronize every other cellular clock in the body—governing when you feel awake, when you

produce hormones, when your immune system peaks, and when you feel sleepy. Disrupted by modern light environments.
→ *See Chapter 2.*

Seed Oils
See Industrial Seed Oils.

Serotonin
A neurotransmitter associated with mood stability, well-being, and calm focus. Approximately 90 percent of the body's serotonin is produced in the gut—by gut cells in interaction with the microbiome. Serotonin is also the direct precursor to melatonin: the body converts serotonin into melatonin as darkness falls. Low serotonin is associated with depression, anxiety, and impulsive eating.
→ *See Chapters 5 and 2.*

Slow-Wave Sleep
See Deep Sleep.

Social Jet Lag
The circadian disruption caused by sleeping significantly different hours on weekends compared to weekdays. If you wake at 6:00 a.m. on weekdays and 9:00 a.m. on weekends, you are shifting your biological clock by three hours—twice a week, every week. The effect on the body is similar to regularly flying across time zones. Associated with metabolic dysfunction, mood disruption, and impaired immune function.
→ *See Chapter 2—Question 9 of the audit.*

Stress Hormones

Primarily cortisol and adrenaline—the hormones released by the adrenal glands in response to stress. Both are designed to prepare the body for immediate physical action. In the modern environment, they are triggered constantly (by screens, emails, noise, and worry) but the physical discharge that should follow never—leaving stress hormones chronically elevated.

→ *See Chapter 3.*

Sympathetic Nervous System

The division of the autonomic nervous system responsible for the fight-or-flight response—the accelerator. It raises heart rate, dilates airways, increases blood glucose, shunts blood to muscles, and suppresses digestion. Its counterpart, the parasympathetic nervous system, is the brake—governing rest, digestion, and repair.

→ *See Chapter 3.*

—T—

Triglycerides

The form in which fat is stored in fat cells and transported in the blood. When you eat more calories than your body needs—particularly from carbohydrates and sugar—the excess is converted into triglycerides and stored. When insulin is low (fasting, sleep, low-carb eating), triglycerides are broken down and used for energy by lipoprotein lipase.

→ *See Chapter 3.*

—U—

Ultra-Processed Food

Food products manufactured through industrial processes and formulated from substances extracted from whole foods—refined starches, hydrogenated oils, added sugars, protein isolates, artificial flavors, colors, and preservatives. They are designed for maximum palatability, shelf stability, and repeat purchase. Generally very low in fiber and micronutrients, and very high in caloric density, industrial seed oils, and additives.

→ *See Chapter 1.*

—V—

Vagus Nerve

The longest nerve in the body, running from the brainstem through the chest and abdomen, connecting the brain to the heart, lungs, and digestive system. The primary highway of the parasympathetic (rest and digest) nervous system. Physical movement—particularly walking—stimulates the vagus nerve, lowering heart rate, reducing cortisol, and shifting the nervous system from fight-or-flight toward rest and recovery.

→ *See Chapter 3.*

Vitamin D

A fat-soluble vitamin that functions as a hormone throughout the body. Produced in the skin when UVB light hits a cholesterol precursor (7-dehydrocholesterol). Regulates calcium

absorption, immune function, gene expression (approximately three thousand genes carry vitamin D response elements), and mental health. Deficiency is widespread—estimated to affect over one billion people globally—primarily because modern life is lived almost entirely indoors.
→ *See Chapter 9.*

Vitamin K2
A fat-soluble vitamin distinct from vitamin K1. Its primary role is to activate proteins that tell calcium where to go in the body—directing it into bone and teeth, and away from soft tissues and arteries. Found in fermented foods (natto, aged cheese) and some animal products. Critically important when supplementing vitamin D3, which increases calcium absorption; without K2, that calcium has no routing signal.
→ *See Chapter 9.*

—Z—

Zinc
A trace mineral essential for immune function, wound healing, protein synthesis, DNA repair, taste, smell, and hormone production. The vitamin D receptor is a zinc-finger protein—meaning it requires zinc in its molecular structure to bind to DNA and carry out vitamin D's genetic functions. Abundant in shellfish (especially oysters), red meat, and organ meats.
→ *See Chapter 9.*

A Final Note

Every term in this book that might give a reader pause is defined here. The goal is simple: no one should ever have to stop and search for a definition while they are reading.

Index

Red Triangle

Workers, Loyalists and Partition – a North of Ireland History

Fearghal Mac Bhloscaidh

VERSO
London • New York

First published by Verso 2026

The publisher and author would like to thank the publications in which earlier version of some chapters first appeared: Ch. 5, 'The Caledon Lockout – Revolution and Counter-revolution in Rural Ulster, 1918–1922', *International Labor and Working-Class History*, Vol. 98, 2020; Ch. 6, 'The Belfast Pogrom and the Interminable Irish Question', *Studi Irlandesi*, Vol. 12, No. 12, 2022; Ch. 7, 'The "Miracle of Coalisland": Class and Sectarianism in the Tyrone Coalfield, 1922–26', *Socialist History*, No. 64, 2024.

The manufacturer's authorised representative in the EU for product safety (GPSR) is LOGOS EUROPE, 9 rue Nicolas Poussin, 17000, La Rochelle, France
contact@logoseurope.eu

1 3 5 7 9 10 8 6 4 2

Verso
UK: 6 Meard Street, London W1F 0EG
US: 207 East 32nd Street, New York, NY 10016
versobooks.com

Verso is the imprint of New Left Books

ISBN-13: 978-1-83674-187-9
ISBN-13: 978-1-83674-189-3 (US EBK)
ISBN-13: 978-1-83674-188-6 (UK EBK)

British Library Cataloguing in Publication Data
A catalogue record for this book is available from the British Library

Library of Congress Cataloging-in-Publication Data
A catalog record for this book is available from the Library of Congress

Typeset in Minion by Hewer Text UK Ltd, Edinburgh
Printed and bound by CPI Group (UK) Ltd, Croydon, CR0 4YY